Praise for
Reversing Gum Disease Naturally

"*Reversing Gum Disease Naturally* emphasizes the blending of the classical and holistic approaches to oral hygienic health care. Sandra Senzon, R.D.H., emphasizes the gentle, natural nurturing of the gingival tissues in order to resist bacterial invasion, and thus maintain your proper gingival health. She also stresses the concept of teeth lasting for a lifetime through enlightened prevention, including proper home care and oral hygiene. This book allows the patient to be an active participant along with healthcare professionals."

—Jay P. Goldsmith, D.M.D.

"*Reversing Gum Disease Naturally* presents techniques and information so that you can reverse already unhealthy states in your mouth or prevent the onset of gum disease. Sandra Senzon enhances patients' oral health through traditional as well as holistic methods."

—Barry Musikant, D.M.D.

"After reading Sandra Senzon's book, there is a ray of hope at the end of the tunnel for all those who suffer from gum disease. We ultimately don't have to lose our natural teeth. Sandra Senzon shows us the many ways in which the mouth is connected to the body, and how, with the use of natural herbal products and proper mechanic techniques, you can reverse gum disease naturally."

—Joseph P. Greer, D.O.S.

REVERSING
GUM DISEASE
NATURALLY

REVERSING GUM DISEASE NATURALLY

A Holistic Home Care Program

Sandra Senzon, R.D.H.

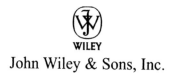

WILEY

John Wiley & Sons, Inc.

Published by John Wiley & Sons, Inc., Hoboken, New Jersey
Published simultaneously in Canada

The information contained in this book is not intended to serve as a replacement
for professional medical advice. Any use of the information in this book is at the
reader's discretion. The author and the publishser specifically disclaim any and all
liability arising directly or indirectly from the use or application of any
information contained in this book. A health care professional should be
consulted regarding your specific situation.

For general information about our other products and services, please contact our
Customer Care Department within the United States at (800) 762-2974, outside
the United States at (317) 572-3993 or fax (317) 572-4002.

Wiley also publishes its books in a variety of electronic formats. Some content
that appears in print may not be available in electronic books. For more
information about Wiley products, visit our web site at www.wiley.com.

Library of Congress Cataloging-in-Publication Data:
Senzon, Sandra.
    Reversing gum disease naturally : a holistic home care program. / Sandra
Senzon.
        p. ; cm.
Includes bibliographical references and index.
        ISBN 0-471-22230-5 (paper)
    1. Gums—Diseases—Alternative treatment. 2. Periodontal
disease—Alternative treatment. 3. Naturopathy.
        [DNLM: 1. Gingival Diseases—therapy—Popular Works. 2. Holistic
Health—Popular Works. 3. Nautropathy—Popular Works. 4. Preventive
Dentistry—methods—Popular Works.   WU 240 S478r 2003]   I. Title.
    RK401 .S46 2003
    617.6'32—dc21   2002153471

To my patients, who have kept me going in trying times, and to the dentists, who have grown to love my style.

Contents

Contents

Contents

Foreword

If you feel that you lack control in the dental office, the problem might be a lack of information. *Reversing Gum Disease Naturally* is an in-depth discussion of the oral cavity and its relationship to the rest of the body, and it is written on a level that both the dental professional and the layperson can understand. In simple terms, Sandra Senzon, R.D.H., increases your dental IQ, which can give you greater control when you work with dental professionals.

I first became acquainted with Sandra, a registered dental hygienist, when she began treating patients in my office on Madison Avenue in New York City. Sandra has been active in clinical treatment since 1977. She has an extensive following of loyal patients who have continued to improve periodontally as a result of her techniques, which are well described in this book. They include natural, nonsurgical periodontal treatments and state-of-the-art cleaning with herbs, coupled with education about hygiene at home and quality dentistry.

The material in this book is up-to-date, practical, and well presented. It encompasses the full scope of conditions of the body and their relationship to the oral cavity. As Sandra puts it, "The mouth is a mirror of the body's health." Sandra has worked tirelessly to put the mouth and body into a natural balance, and she draws on over twenty-five years of experience in treating patients' gums and in presenting a practical and natural approach to her work. This informative book is for all those who are concerned about the health of their mouth.

— Mitchell Charnas, D.M.D.

Acknowledgments

I give special thanks to my publisher, who saw merit in this book, and to my agent, Jeff Herman, who believed in me. My children, Eric and Bari, have always been there with a special kind of support. Thanks also to the artist, Aaron. All of you are wonderful.

I also thank myself for having the courage to write about this topic in a humanistic manner!

Introduction

Have you been told that you have periodontal disease? Do you dread losing your teeth? My book will guide you to the *truth* about gum disease. *Reversing Gum Disease Naturally* is packed with information you need to help you keep your natural teeth. Treatment of gum disease does not have to be the painful experience that unfortunately has been for some of my patients who have been treated by hygienists practicing other techniques. Reading this book will acquaint you with oral hygiene and help you learn what you can do to keep healthy gums and teeth.

Gum tissue is a covering around the roots of our teeth that is in great need of massage and cleansing. We abuse our mouths regularly by grinding and clenching our teeth, and by eating foods with sugar and spices. Many of us also eat sticky, adhesive-type foods. At my hygiene center, I work with natural herbs that feed the gum tissue in healthy ways. Ninety percent of the cure for gum disease entails not only patient education but motivation in terms of dental hygiene home care. Proper instruction will allow and foster corrective home care maintenance.

Articles and advertisements on plaque and tartar talk about bacteria invading the structures of the mouth. But what about the fragile tissue that holds these bacteria? If we condition gum tissue on a regular basis, we would not have a holding pocket for food and bacteria to sit next to the tooth and bone! Bacteria will always be present in the body and mouth, but we can learn to nurture our mouth and gently bring it to a healthy state.

When I began my career twenty-six years ago, I saw that people had tremendous problems with the loss of adult teeth. Even though I was instructed to teach patients to brush and floss, I saw that brushing and flossing were not enough. I noticed that the patients' gum tissue seemed stretched and loose around crowns and bridges, areas where there is much irritation to the surrounding tissue due to crown margins and materials used for crowns and bridges. As I continued to evaluate the condition of these patients, I saw the need for greater tissue-hygiene control.

As a dedicated practitioner, I researched and evaluated products from all over the world that can help heal these conditions, and I brought them back home to offer to my own patients. I developed and marketed a "home care kit" containing a toothbrush, baking soda toothpaste, rubber tip, mirror, and instructional brochure. This kit has been promoted at the International Gift Show and at dental trade shows. As a result of this, I have been interviewed by many trade magazines. I continue to get a great deal of publicity for my efforts, and this has led me to travel all over the world seeking the best products that are available.

I now have a Tooth Spa on Madison Avenue in New York City, where my colleagues and I work on gums as well as clean and whiten teeth. I had a book published, *The Hygiene Professional: A Partner in Dentistry,* to help train other dental hygienists to work in the same fashion. After the evolution of the Tooth Spa came the creation of a character aptly named the Tooth Fairy. Using this character, I initiated the first dental hygiene educational show on cable television, called *The Tooth Fairy Show.* I have written a series of five children's books, *Tooth Fairy City,* to help motivate and educate children, and have even lectured in hospitals and schools dressed as the Tooth Fairy!

After reading my book, you will have an excellent chance of keeping your teeth and gums healthy, and you will not be misled by the "business" of dentistry. The information contained in this book will help you work better with your dental professional, and also to control the maintenance of your mouth by yourself. Your teeth and gums will let you know how they are feeling, and as you become acquainted with various problems, you will be able to work on them as they arise. Whatever you do, do not wait until the problems become so severe that they are more difficult to reverse.

PART I

ABOUT GUM DISEASE

Part I will describe gum disease and its onset. In these chapters, you will get a new and broader understanding of your mouth and how it is a mirror of your body. Stress, fear, and pain are major causes of gum disease, and in Part I, healing modalities will be discussed on how to reduce stress, pain, and fear.

Read on, and you will be delighted to see that the mouth is connected to the total body. You will begin to *reverse gum disease naturally!*

1

Gum Disease

Its Signs, and the First Steps Toward Healing

Understanding Gum Disease

With increased awareness of periodontal disease and a greater selection of dental hygiene products available, why is gum disease the most commonly diagnosed health problem among today's American adult population, affecting approximately 40 million people? Since this disease of the mouth has a destructive nature, it is important that you follow the guidelines described in this book to help begin the healing process. People have been losing their teeth as part of the aging process; however, with routine cleanings and good home care, we can all keep our natural teeth. If you exercise preventive care, it is not unreasonable to expect your teeth and gums to last a lifetime.

To understand gum disease in simple terms, think of your teeth rooted in bone the way a plant is rooted in soil. If the soil supporting the plant begins to erode, the plant will

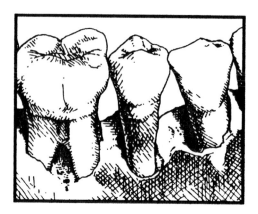

Tooth rooted in bone.

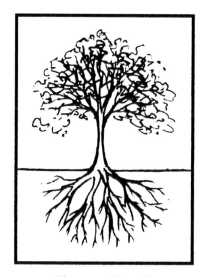

Plant rooted in soil.

loosen and bend. The same thing can happen with your teeth. If the bone that supports the teeth in their sockets begins to erode, the teeth will loosen and fall out.

The first stage of periodontal disease is called *gingivitis:* *gingiv* (gum tissue) and *itis* (inflammation). This initial stage is characterized by loose, swollen, tender, and/or bleeding gums. The loose, flabby gum tissue allows pockets to form between the teeth and the gum tissue—pockets in which food debris can collect and harmful bacteria can multiply. The bacteria may then attack the neighboring jawbone, causing it to erode. When bone loss has occurred, the disease has progressed to the second stage. This is known as *periodontitis,* and is classified as early, moderate, or advanced, depending on the degree of bone destruction.

What causes gingivitis? Gingivitis is a bacterial infection of the gum tissue. Bacteria live in plaque, a sticky film that accumulates on your teeth every day. Plaque needs to be removed by proper oral home care. If it is not removed properly, the toxins in the plaque will cause the gums to get irritated and infected. Plaque left on the teeth and not disrupted by brushing and flossing will calcify and turn into *calculus* (commonly called "tartar"). Brushing and flossing cannot remove calculus; it must be removed by a professional. Calculus found caked on the roots of diseased teeth, in addition to containing bacterial toxins, is a mechanical irritant to the soft tissue.

Signs of Disease

There are many signs that indicate the presence of gum disease. They can include:

- *Halitosis, or bad breath.* An end product of this disease process and tissue breakdown is very often mouth malodor, or *halitosis,* commonly called "bad breath." Although halitosis is a common symptom of periodontal disease, it may be caused by other health problems or conditions as well, such as gastritis (acid stomach). If your breath is sour in the morning, it might be due to dehydration or loss of saliva during sleep. And certain allergies can leave a bacterial mucous that mixes with your saliva and causes bad breath. Many medications also have side effects that can leave you with bad breath. Therefore, you should seek out a professional for a diagnosis of what is causing the halitosis.

    However, to determine if you have halitosis, cup your hands over your mouth and breathe out. Then smell. If you detect an odor, then you probably have bad breath. Or ask your spouse or a close friend to inform you if you have this problem. To determine if the halitosis is originating from your mouth, try smelling your dental floss after you have used it. If the floss has a foul odor, the halitosis is probably emanating from your teeth and gums.

- *Malpositioned teeth.* Another warning sign of periodontal disease is loose and malpositioned teeth. Teeth will move out of place due to bone loss. If your teeth are moving out of position and seem to overlap, or if gaps are forming between your teeth, this may be a warning sign that you have gum disease. There are other reasons for loose teeth, such as a fractured root, so do seek a professional to obtain a proper diagnosis. Do not try to diagnose the condition yourself!

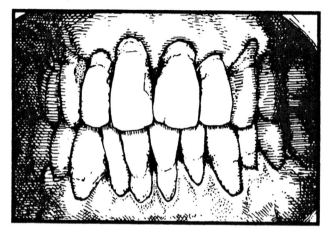

Receding gums.

- *Receding gums.* Have you ever heard the expression, "long in the tooth"? This is used to describe receding gums, or gums that are "backing away" from the teeth. The condition is the result of gum and bone loss and subsequent root exposure, thus giving the tooth a longer appearance. Sensitivity can occur as well, because the root does not have an enamel covering. Enamel covers the crowns of your teeth and acts as a protective covering.
- *Bleeding gums.* Do your gums bleed when you brush your teeth? Bleeding around your gums is an important indication of periodontal disease and is often the first sign you may notice. Bleeding, as well as inflammation and irritation of the gums, may also signal other medical problems, so do not ignore these signs. Seek a professional opinion. Such bleeding also can be a result of

the gum tissue drying out. This can occur if you wear braces or have other problems that keep your lips from closing over your teeth. Allergies may block the nasal passages, leaving you no choice but to breathe through your mouth. The result of mouth breathing, rather than breathing through your nose with your mouth closed, may be gingivitis. An open mouth can cause the tissue to dry out and become loose and irritated. Or, if you have allergies and your saliva has a lot of excess bacteria and mucous, the fragile gum tissue can become infected. People who suffer from postnasal drip have a great deal of mucus in the saliva, and this causes irritated gums.

- *Gum abscesses.* A gum abscess can be another sign of gum disease. If an area of your mouth appears to have a swelling or a lump above the tooth, then you may

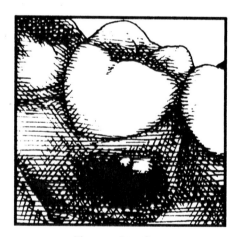

Abscessed tooth.

well have a gum abscess. The invasive bacteria within the abscess will eat away at the supportive bone. The onset of gum disease can begin with just one abscess on one tooth. Bacteria will eat away at the bone surrounding the tooth, resulting in less support to the tooth and ultimately in tooth loss if not properly cared for. An abscess does not necessarily have pain associated with it, but you may have an additional problem originating in the nerve, which will cause pain.

Gum disease is insidious and can progress without your knowledge. Any early signs of this disease, as described above, need your immediate attention. If you lose bone, which roots your teeth into their sockets, your teeth will lack support and will loosen or fall out. Bone, ligaments, and gum tissue all support the positioning of the teeth. But diseased conditions of our body can be reversed as long as we do not deny that they exist.

The History of Gum Disease

Luckily, many dentists have been true pioneers in the prevention of tooth loss and have helped create the techniques and instruments for scaling teeth that are used today.

Knowledge of gum disease dates back as far as 1746, when Dr. Pierre Fauchard, a surgeon-dentist who is known as the father of modern dentistry, wrote a paper titled *Le Chirurgien Dentiste* that described gum disease. Dr. Fauchard advised patients to wash out their mouths with tepid water after having cleaned their teeth. After they rinsed, he advised patients to rub the teeth from below upward, and from above downward—outside and inside—with a little sponge dipped in water. He also claimed it was good to use a half-round toothpick to remove what he called the "fur" that collects on or between the teeth and gums during the night. His advice to remove this sticky film with a toothpick was very advanced for his time, and his ideas presaged today's use of picks to scale teeth.

In 1845 Dr. John Hankey Riggs was the first to call attention to gum disease in America. Periodontal disease thus became known as "Riggs disease." Few professionals currently refer to gum disease as Riggs disease, however. Today's terms are: gum disease, periodontal disease, or gingivitis. My own approach is much the same as his: to treat the condition as a curable disease by cleaning the pockets surrounding the teeth. With a thorough cleaning, the bacteria and toxins are removed from between the teeth and surrounding bone, thus reversing gum disease.

Dr. Riggs is given credit for designing scalers and curettes—instruments that we still use today to remove the hardened stone (tartar) from the roots of our teeth and the diseased layer of granular (thickened diseased tissue) that sits next to the tartar. The roots of our teeth are not straight up and down, but curve at angles under the gum tissue. Thus the scalers and curettes were designed with contra-angles (curved angles) to conform to the roots and remove any material in the pockets. A dental cleaning using these instruments is the most important preventive treatment for periodontal disease.

One of the first dentists in America to establish a *preventive* dental practice was Dr. David Smith of Philadelphia in 1894. Prophylactic services (cleaning of teeth), although

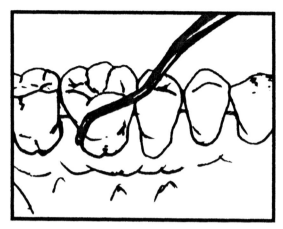

Clinical instrument with curved angles.

beneficial to patients, were time-consuming, and so reduced the amount of time dentists were able to allocate to restorative treatment. Thus there were fewer dentists back then who performed preventive care. Most were *restorative* dentists, who focused on fixing the nonregenerative enamel and dentin, the hardened materials of our teeth. Dr. Alfred C. Fones, another pioneer, believed that training auxiliary personnel to provide prophylactic care was an efficient solution to this problem. Dental hygiene thus can be traced back to Dr. Fones, as he felt there should be a separation between restorative care and gum disease, and he was the first to initiate a program for dental hygiene. A *dental hygienist* is a licensed professional who cleans away the tartar (hardened plaque) from the teeth and roots under the gums. Dr. Fones created a school for dental hygiene in Bridgeport, Connecticut, in 1898.

It was understood even then that not enough emphasis was put on educating children and teaching them the importance of proper oral hygiene. It was known as far back as 1898 that a clean tooth would not decay. So dental hygiene became an important profession in helping adults and children prevent adult tooth decay and tooth loss. The dental hygienist would clean teeth, educate and motivate the patients in home care, and then recommend treatment for restorative care by the dentist. The dental hygienist's role was an important one—even more than it is today—for there were fewer dentists at that time.

In 1939 Dr. A. W. Byran tried to make the dental profession aware of causative factors in gum disease and attempted to have the profession focus on prevention and diagnosis, rather than only on the symptoms of the disease. He argued against drug treatment, maintaining that unless the drugs were directed at a specific site of infection, they were not treating the condition scientifically. He was also against the surgical removal of unattached tissue because it did not address the cause and only dealt with symptoms.

Dr. Byran and Dr. Riggs had more insight into the subject of the reversal of gum disease naturally than many gum specialists (periodontists) do today, as cutting away at diseased and unattached tissue is still widely practiced. While surgical removal of gum tissue instantly shrinks the pocket collecting bacteria, the tissue remains thinner at a higher point on the tooth. And if the periodontist does not address the cause and motivate the person to practice proper home care and oral hygiene, the condition can appear again and cause breakdown in a more vulnerable area.

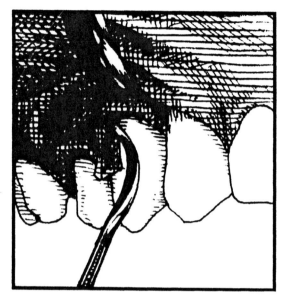

Surgical removal of a pocket.

The Natural Process of Healing: How It Begins

The natural reversal process of gum disease starts with proper instrumentation in the dental office. If you have gum disease, the first step is to go to a dentist's office for a cleaning. Dental hygienists and dentists are trained specifically to treat the gums and provide proper cleanings to help eliminate the hardened material or tartar that attaches to the tooth and root structure. It is important for the hygienist or the dentist to do a thorough cleaning and to work with hand instruments (see chapter 6) for these procedures. Many offices today rely on high-tech equipment such as the ultrasonic scaler and the Prophy Jet. But focused therapeutic healing can also come from the practitioner, traveling through the hands, through the instruments, and into the patient's mouth. High-tech instruments, such as the sonic scaler (high-speed ultrasonic tartar remover), can be an obstacle to this kind of healing. (Therapeutic healing will be discussed in chapter 6.)

Your mouth may require more than one cleaning; it all depends on the severity of your condition. If your mouth is in the second or third stage of periodontal disease, then you might have to return for three or four treatments. A return for maintenance can be as frequent as four or five times a year. After a root planing treatment (a cleaning of the roots so that healing can take place), the tissue will begin to reattach to the root and return to a healthy state. After the removal of tartar, you can use a natural process at home to heal the tissue (this will be discussed in chapter 9). This is equally as important as getting a thorough professional cleaning. Proper home care can help speed up the results of the gum treatments that are done in the dental office.

After you have root planing and scaling in the dentist's office, you will discover that your gum tissue will be sore and fragile. So go home and use distilled warm water with sea salt or an herbal rinse, preferably Dr. Vogel's Bioforce (Dentaforce), to enable the tissue to heal. Rinse your mouth frequently and also massage the tissue with a soft brush. Such soreness tells us it is important to work in a slow and careful fashion. You would not beat up on a wound that was raw and new. So keep in mind that all healing is a gentle process and takes time.

These are the six steps that will happen when you go in for a holistic cleaning or gum treatment.

1. The dentist or periodontist reviews the patient's condition and charts the pockets with a periodontal probe (Pockets over 4 mm are considered a prerequisite for gum disease.) Charting of the teeth allows professionals to make note of their evaluation of your mouth. They will also document crowns and bridges, missing teeth, teeth that show broken fillings, and teeth that have decay and need fillings or root canals.
2. The dentist suggests a treatment plan. Since everyone heals differently, it may take longer for some people, and they may need several appointments.
3. The professional provides cleanings, preferably with hand instrumentation. Ideally, an instrument is dipped in oreganol (oil of oregano), olive oil, or clove oil, and then in echinacea toothpaste or another natural toothpaste. The oreganol or clove oil acts as a lubricant and natural numbing agent. The echinacea or natural toothpaste feeds the new cells of the gum.
4. The patient uses a rinse, preferably herbal, to rid the mouth of disease.
5. The professional conducts a brush massage of the gums to soothe the irritated tissue and teach the patient the therapeutic methods of massaging the gums. At this point, the patient rinses again.
6. The professional provides a review of home care instruction. The patient is often given a package that usually contains toothpaste (herbal or baking soda is preferred) for cleansing and healing of the tissue,

mouth rinse, toothbrush, and perhaps selected herbal products. The professional then advises the patient on how to start caring for the gums at home.

How to Start Caring for Your Gums at Home

Gum tissue is connected to the bone by fibers. You can achieve reattachment of these gum fibers by using a gentle massaging stroke with a soft brush. So, using the side of a small-headed, soft toothbrush that has a dab of herbal toothpaste on it, gently massage the tissue with a shimmying side-to-side stroke.

Such massage stimulates circulation, which aids healing in the gum tissue. Using a massage stroke with a soft brush will help you bring the healing blood cells of the gums to the surface. It is the healing cells of the gums that will help to reattach gum tissue to the tooth. Think of the skin on your

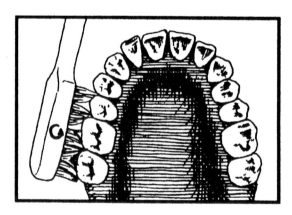

Brush massage.

face. If you massage the skin on your face and create more circulation, then you are more likely to get a healthier and tighter appearance to your skin. The gum tissue is similar to the skin on your face in that both need proper products and massage. In Chinese medicine, natural blood-building tonics such as dong quai improve circulation. This can bring a healthy blood flow and stimulation to the gum tissue, and balance the female hormonal chemistry, which has a direct correlation to the health of our gum tissue.

If the gum tissue feels too sore when you first practice brush massage, then just proceed by rinsing frequently. In a day or two, when the tissue heals, you can begin massaging the gums again in order to bring the healing blood cells to the surface.

Do not rush the process, or you will irritate the gums and cause more harm than good. If your gums bleed and you are frightened to work on them because you think you may make the condition worse, seek the advice of a professional. Bleeding gums can be a sign that there is disease still present. However, with a gentle massage, the healing blood cells generally will surface to start reversing the disease naturally. Salt water and herbal rinses will help soothe any irritated tissue. Also, start taking a multiple vitamin B complex daily along with vitamin C. This will help in the natural healing process of your gums. If you feel you are under a lot of stress (which is a major cause of gum disease), take a multiple vitamin with zinc. Keep the gum pockets clean and gently floss. If you find that flossing is too hard at this point and causes pain, then work only with oral rinses of herbs and salt. In a few days, when your gums feel stronger, you can return to flossing.

As your mouth continues to recover from the treatment it received in the dental office, recognize that the foods you eat after root planing should not be too hot or too cold. Think of your gums as you would your skin: if you were to put ice or a hot substance on your skin, you would then notice irritation. The same condition can arise in your mouth. Another important suggestion is to stay away from spices when you are trying to heal your gum tissue. If you had a wound on your hand, you would not apply spices to the surface of the wound. The same applies to your gums. So it is best to eat bland foods while your gums are healing.

Miso (Japanese soy) soup is very soothing to the gum tissue, and you can feel the effects after drinking it. Avoid eating fruit with a lot of vitamin C after gum treatments. While the fruit may provide the proper nutrients to strengthen the gum tissue, the acids from the juices that come in direct contact with the gums may irritate the healing tissue. Juices that are very acidic, such as orange or grapefruit, are not recommended immediately after a cleaning. Biting into an orange or other citrus fruit will irritate the gum tissue. Also, try to stay away from hard nuts and candy. Candy and sugar turn to acid in the mouth, and this will irritate the gum tissue. After a few days, if you want orange juice, sip the juice through a straw.

Such nurturing of the tissue will accelerate the reattachment of the gum fibers to the tooth. The soreness and pain should lessen with time. Pain in the gum tissue feels like a dull ache and will diminish in a day or two after a professional scaling and root planing. Healing is a natural process that can be accelerated through the power of positive thoughts. If you are confident and understand the natural process of healing that is taking place in your mouth, then you will achieve faster results.

Follow these other guidelines:

- **Sleep well:** Sleep will allow the immune system to be restored.
- **Eat a proper diet:** Food plays an important role in healing the mouth and body.
- **Use vitamin therapy:** Vitamin B complex with C and magnesium is helpful; always remember, diet is most important.
- **Drink soothing liquids:** Foods that heal include miso soup and chicken soup.
- **Rinse frequently:** Sea salt and herbal rinses soothe the gum tissue.
- **Massage the gum tissue:** Use an herbal toothpaste—herbs soothe the gum tissue and nurture new cells.
- **Oxygenate:** Breathe deeply—take in lots of oxygen.
- **Think positively:** Mind over matter—the mind operates the healing process.

2

The Mouth Is a Mirror of the Body

Diseases of the Body and Medications That Can Affect Your Gums

The mouth mirrors certain conditions of the body, and doctors as well as dental professionals have discovered that some diseases can also affect the mouth and gums. In other words, gum irritation may be a secondary symptom of a diseased condition in your body. Sometimes the mouth is the first part of the body to reflect the body's diseased condition.

In addition, stress and diet can wreak havoc in your mouth. The effects of stress will be discussed in chapter 3.

Conditions of the Body That Cause Gum Disease

Diabetes

Conditions such as diabetes can appear as gum disease and be the causative factor of the problem. Diabetes is a chronic degenerative disease caused by a lack of the hormone insulin. Insulin is essential for the proper metabolism of blood sugar. Excessive glucose (blood sugar) in the body's system is toxic. People with diabetes have abnormally high carbohydrate and sugar in their diets. Gum disease and dental problems are more prevalent in patients with diabetes and excessive glucose levels. People with diabetes also have a tendency to have bad breath due to excess acid in their systems. It is well known by dental professionals that patients with diabetes have dry mouths, and that less oxygen is consumed by their system. The lack of oxygen to the mouth can cause the gum tissue to dry out and loosen. Loose gum tissue can lead to pockets that then become a holding place for food and bacteria, and the bacteria under the gum can eat away the bone. In addition, people with diabetes have difficulty healing; therefore, even a scraping of the gum can lead to a sore, infected abscess.

People who have diabetes can easily acquire abscesses on their gums and usually have noticeable changes of the mucous membranes in their mouth. A condition called angular chelitis can develop, which appears as cracks in the corners of the mouth. This is common for people with diabetes.

Remedies

- See your dental hygienist frequently for cleanings.
- Ask your doctor about regulating your diet, so that you are less prone to excessive blood sugar levels.
- Drink healing foods, in particular, juices that can reduce the acids in your mouth. The juice from string beans, parsley, cucumber, celery, and watercress can reduce acid-mouth. Another suggestion is to combine

carrots, celery, parsley, spinach, and broccoli in a blender. Use three or four carrots with stems, four or five stems each of celery and broccoli, and a few sprigs of parsley along with a handful of spinach. Process, and have one or two glasses of this a day. Juice made from all these ingredients will help "cool down" the gum tissue that has become "heated up" from acids in the mouth. Blueberries are also a smart food choice, as they create a more alkaline environment in the mouth.

Menstruation

Women often show signs of gum problems during menstruation. This is because the monthly cycle brings on various hormonal changes among the hypothalamus, the pituitary gland, and the ovaries. At the beginning of each cycle, estrogen causes a thickening of the lining of the uterus (the endometrium) with blood; the cervical fluid is released, resulting in menstruation.

The mouth also releases fluid, and bleeding gums may appear before, during, and sometimes after menstruation. Hormonal changes also affect gum tissue, leaving the gums soft and spongy. Have you noticed that around the time of your period your toothbrush becomes red? Don't get scared; it is a natural process. I have observed that when my female patients have abnormally soft, spongy gum tissue, they are either menstruating or about to menstruate. Your immune system also is affected by hormonal changes. A weakened area in your mouth may become even weaker at this time. You also may notice an area in your mouth that bothers you during menstruation, and then after your period cycle it seems to be fine.

Remedies

- Massage the gums with a soft brush, which brings blood flow to them.
- Brush with a cleanser such as baking soda, which will also neutralize the acids in your mouth. Baking soda is not abrasive and can help keep the space between the teeth and gums clean.
- Rinse with sea salt.
- If you are premenstrual or have your menses, eat fresh fruit, vegetables, whole grains, nuts, seeds, and fish.

Oral Contraceptives and Pregnancy

Inflammation of the gums is common in women who take oral contraceptives and in women who are pregnant. The gum tissues become swollen and engorged with blood. Birth control pills work by introducing high levels of estrogen and progesterone into the body, to fool it into thinking it is pregnant.

If you are pregnant and notice a swelling or lump on the gums surrounding one or more teeth, you probably have what is known as "a pregnancy tumor." This lesion is not really a tumor but a local area of granulated (thickened) tissue. Pregnancy tumors disappear after your pregnancy ceases.

Remedies

- Massage the gum tissue with a soft brush, which will help reduce inflammation.
- Use baking soda toothpaste or baking soda straight out of the box, as this can reduce swelling. Baking soda is

an antacid that can balance the pH of your mouth, leaving it less prone to gum disease and tooth decay.
- Use sea salt rinses to help reduce swollen tissue.
- Consult your gynecologist about a proper diet.
- See your dental hygienist frequently for cleanings.

Menopause

Women who enter menopause go through hormonal changes. Usually there is a lack of estrogen and progesterone, which causes osteoporosis. Osteoporosis is the thinning and loss of bone structure in the body. In the mouth there can be a form of osteoporosis leading to bone loss surrounding the teeth. The bone supports the teeth and holds them in their sockets. New bone is made by osteoblast (bone-building) cells, and old bone is restored by osteoblasts. However, estrogen in the body reduces osteoblasts, causing bone resorption. The role of progesterone is to stimulate the osteoblasts that aid in new bone formation. Thus progesterone is very important in stimulating new bone growth. Hormones play an important role in gum disease and can be the precursor to the condition.

Remedies: Seek advice from your gynecologist regarding hormone replacement in menopause.

Prior to and during menopause, certain foods can help eliminate your symptoms of gum disease. Papaya, for example, contains phytoestrogen, which can be added to your diet to help increase estrogen in your body. Estrogen levels can increase with the intake of certain foods such as soybeans and soy products such as tofu, miso, and boiled beans. Phytoestrogen is also found in apples, carrots, yams, green beans, peas, potatoes, red beans, brown rice, whole wheat, rye, and sesame seeds. Flaxseeds and other seeds have some estrogen potential. Phytoestrogens are similar but not identical to the estrogen produced by the body. Phytoestrogens are plant-derived compounds, and are more natural than the prescribed drugs on the market. If you notice that your skin is dry, take flaxseed or pumpkin seed.

Additional remedies

- **Herbs:** Use rosemary or oreganol (oil of oregano), which are both helpful in the prevention of gum shrinkage.
- **Hormone replacement:** To regulate the hormone levels in your body, seek a physician's advice.
- **Diet:** Soybeans, tofu, miso, boiled beans, apples, carrots, yams, green beans, peas, potatoes, red beans, brown rice, whole wheat, rye, and sesame seeds are good. Flaxseed acts as a lubricant and will help prevent dry skin and gums from receding. Your gums are similar to your skin, and you want to moisturize your gum tissue as you would your skin.

Anemia

Anemia is a disease in which people have reduced red blood cells, which can result in poor circulation. The blood in patients with anemia lacks iron and carries less oxygen to the tissues, and this causes periodontal problems. The symptoms of anemia are extreme fatigue, weakness, confusion and loss of concentration, pale skin, rapid heartbeat, feeling cold, sadness, and depression. Getting oxygen to the tissue is important for healthy gums, and the lack of it reduces resistance to infection.

Anemia is most prevalent in women who are menstruating or pregnant; and African Americans are prone to getting sickle cell anemia. If you have this condition, you should know that you can have serious calcium loss. The chances of gum disease are great for anyone who has this condition, because calcium is needed for strong teeth and bones. If you have a shortage of calcium, it may affect the supportive bone structure that holds the teeth in their sockets.

Remedies: Seaweed, which may be purchased in health food stores, is the best source of iron. Liver is another good source of iron. Pumpkin seeds and sesame seeds are also good choices for people who are anemic. Apples contain substances that help the body absorb the iron in foods such as eggs and liver. Cherries are high in iron and are an excellent blood builder. Anemia is most prevalent in women who are menstruating or pregnant. Iron is deficient in these conditions, and it is suggested that you seek advice from your physician about taking supplements. And if your gum tissue is spongy and loose, see your dental professional for a good cleaning.

Herpes Simplex Virus

Herpes simplex is an inflammatory viral disease that manifests itself as ulcers in the mouth and gingival tissues. The gums can become inflamed, especially in the region of the ulcers. If you have a severe occurrence of the virus, then you should seek medical advice to see if there are other underlying factors causing this condition. Herpes simplex can be chronic and latent, returning later in life. The gums can become inflamed, especially in the regions of the ulcers.

Remedies: Seek medical advice. Bed rest is important. Drink plenty of fluids, and stay away from juices that contain acid, such as grapefruit juice and orange juice.

Dermatitis

Dermatitis is a diseased condition that appears as inflammation of the skin. The gum tissue is much like the skin on your face and shares similar histologic (cellular structure) characteristics. Diseases affecting your skin are lichen planus, candidiasis, psoriasis, pemphigus vulgaris, and pemphigoid.

Lichen planus is a chronic disease related to the immune system, often affecting people in middle age. It affects the mucous membranes of the mouth. You may see a white lacy line on the gingiva (gum tissue). You may be prone to plaque retention on the teeth and therefore develop gingivitis.

Remedies: If you have lichen planus, seek medical advice. Topical steroids can be useful in controlling flare-ups. There is no cure for this problem.

Candidiasis is produced by candida, a fungal yeast infection. It is also referred to as thrush or acute pseudomembranous candidiasis. The roof of your mouth and cheeks are covered with white patches that when wiped off, leave a very sensitive, reddened, ulcerative area. This condition can cause more plaque retention and poor oral hygiene conditions, thus creating a severe gum problem.

Remedies: See your physician to have him or her suggest antifungal agents, which can be either topical or systemic.

Psoriasis is a chronic condition that causes a sloughing off of cells. It is often found on the elbows, knees, or other joints, and on the scalp. Psoriasis also can affect the fingernails and the gums and oral cavity. It may leave the gums loose and irritated. Psoriasis, when aggravated, can be itchy and flaky, and a source of great annoyance to the person who has it.

Remedies: A high-protein/low-fat diet can help in controlling the condition. Eating fats and sugars aggravates psoriasis, so it is best to eat lots of raw fruits and vegetables. Cucumbers, celery, and grapefruit, which are known as blood-cooling foods, are extremely good for people with psoriasis. Seek medical advice as well.

Pemphigus affects elderly people, and women more frequently than men. The skin and mucous membranes as well as the gingiva are affected. A reddening of the tissue occurs, which can cause the gums to recede.

Remedies: Seek professional advice. Topical steroids may be necessary.

Pemphigoid is a lesion most common in women beyond middle age. It can affect the oral mucous. It may be a cause of irritation to the gingiva.

Remedies: Seek professional advice. Physicians are most likely to prescribe steroids.

Alcoholism

Alcohol abuse affects the liver. Liver damage may develop into hepatitis or cirrhosis, a chronic inflammatory disease of the liver. Excessive alcohol use also affects the cardiovascular and nervous systems. Oral effects shown in alcoholics include bleeding gums and easy bruising. Individuals who drink excessively usually have poor oral hygiene habits.

Remedies: Have professional cleanings frequently. Take vitamins and try to eat properly. Drink plenty of water and reduce your alcohol consumption. Seek counseling for help in reducing alcohol abuse.

Cancer of the Head and Neck

Cancer of the head and neck can cause gum problems and excessive bleeding. If you have been treated with chemotherapy, you will notice that your gums will bleed easily and you may also be prone to infection. If you have been undergoing radiation treatment, you may find that your mouth is always dry. This condition is called "xerostomia." Dry mouth can cause more plaque retention and make your teeth prone to decay, especially if your gums have receded to the point where the roots are exposed.

Remedies: Have frequent cleanings. Eat a balanced diet and drink more fluids. If you find that you are suffering from dry mouth, there are supplements you can purchase in the drugstore that act as saliva and moisturize the oral cavity. You can purchase Biotine products in health food stores; a mouthwash and toothpaste are available specifically for dry mouth. You can also use baking soda chewing gum, which enhances the flow of saliva and helps neutralize the acids that are prevalent in dry mouth.

HIV

AIDS is defined as acquired immune deficiency syndrome, a severe condition that is different from any other disease because it has no constant specific symptoms. People with HIV infection or AIDS have oral manifestations that appear as inflamed gum tissue and severely inflamed mucous tissue. These individuals can also have abnormalities such as herpes appearing in the mouth, leukoplakia (a whitish patch found on the cheek), and precancerous lesions. People with AIDS are more prone to gingivitis, a reddening of the gum at the tooth margin.

Patients who have AIDS are also prone to getting thrush or candidiasis, a white patch that is usually found on the palate (roof of the mouth). Patients with AIDS also are more likely to have acute necrotizing ulcerative gingivitis (ANUG). With ANUG, a person suffers severe pain in the region of the mouth and has a characteristic, unpleasant mouth odor. There is spontaneous bleeding, and sometimes severe bleeding in the gums.

Remedies: See a dentist or hygienist. Have routine cleanings, and use echinacea toothpaste to nurture the gum tissue. Use aloe to soothe your irritated gums (apply at night only).

Leukemia and Other Diseases

The oral cavity can be a diagnostic indicator for many diseases of the immune system. The lymphocytes (white blood cells, or disease-fighting cells) are the key cells of the immune system. Systemic diseases characterized by reduced host defense include diabetes and Down's syndrome. They are usually accompanied by severe gum disease. Leukemia is another disease that shows up in the gum tissue. In certain forms of leukemia, there is increased susceptibility to infection and periodontal disease. Gum disease is a problem because of the immunosuppression associated with the disease. In certain forms of leukemia, such as myeloblastic leukemia, gingival enlargement occurs as a result of the leukemia cells in the gum tissue.

Remedies: Seek professional guidance. Develop good oral hygiene at home and clean your mouth frequently. Eat softer foods, chew your foods carefully, and drink fluids while you are eating. Have frequent cleanings by your dentist or hygienist; and at home use herbal rinses, keep your mouth clean with baking soda or sea salt, and massage the gums with oreganol (two or three drops on top of an herbal toothpaste).

Medications and Their Effects on Gum Disease

You may be unaware that certain medications can cause changes to your gum tissue and promote gum disease. The most common of these are antiseizure medications taken for epilepsy. Dilantin, for example, is a drug that can create gingival overgrowth, which has the appearance of thickened tissue and loosened gums. Antidepressants such as Paxil, Elavil, and Zoloft create gingival overgrowth and swellings throughout the mouth. Studies have shown that these changes take place on a cellular level and create a more dense tissue. Another drug that causes overgrowth to gum tissue is cyclosporine, used for immunosuppression in people who have had transplants and people with multiple sclerosis.

If you have overgrowth of tissue and are taking antiseizure medication such as Dilantin, or are taking other drugs that may be causing this condition, it is important that

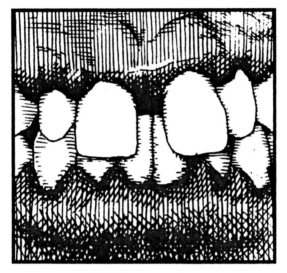

Gingival overgrowth.

you have frequent oral cleanings and that you establish a good oral hygiene regimen (see chapter 6). The thickened, swollen tissues become a greater holding site for plaque and bacteria.

Overgrowth of gum tissue and candidiasis can also be caused by prolonged use of antibiotics, which reduce the body's defense mechanisms by stimulating immunosuppressants. This condition is characterized by a thick white mucous covering on the tongue. Patients with this condition may have more plaque because they have pain from the condition and therefore cannot brush their teeth easily.

It is important that you try to control the problem first. Once this is accomplished, it will be easier to clean your mouth and rid it of plaque. Use natural rinses such as

Bioforce echinacea mouthwash and other herbal rinses found in health food stores. There are rinses that can be prescribed by your dentist or medical doctor to help you with prolonged antibiotic therapy condition.

Lastly, many drugs can create xerostomia (dry mouth), including:

- Anticholinergics, such as atropine, scopolamine, and propantheline
- Antihypertensives, such as guanethidine (Ismelin) and clonidine (Catapres)
- Antihistamines, such as diphenhydramine (Benadryl) and chlorphenermine (Chlortrimeton)
- Antipsychotics, such as chlorpromazine (Thorazine), promazine (Sparine), and thioridazine (Mellaril)
- Amphetamines and narcotics, such as meperidine (Demerol) and morphine
- Anticonvulsants, such as lithium and carbamazepine (Tegretol)
- Antidepressants and anti-anxiety agents, such as Paxil, Elavil, and Zoloft
- Muscle relaxants, such as Norflex and Flexeril
- Diuretics, such as hydrochlorothiazide

Ask your physician if the drugs that you are taking can be the cause of your gum problems. In many of my patients who have thickened saliva and dry mouth, I find that these conditions have been caused by medications. If I have been seeing a patient frequently, and I have not noticed these symptoms before, or they were not recorded on the medical history, I ask the patient if he or she is taking any medication. Dry mouth can cause gum irritation, and the loose gum tissue becomes a greater holding site for bacteria and infected gums.

Remedies: Seek professional advice. Also get over-the-counter saliva replacements, such as Biotine or Arm and Hammer baking soda chewing gum, which will moisturize your mouth. Frequent professional cleanings also help. At home, use frequent herbal mouth rinses to moisturize your mouth.

The Role Tobacco Plays

Tobacco use is an important risk factor in periodontal disease. It is likely that tobacco suppresses certain components of the immune system. Impaired neutrophil (white blood cell) function, induced by the use of tobacco-containing products, appears to have an impact on the gums. In fact, smoking can irritate and stretch the gum tissue. Smoking also suppresses the immune system, leaving you open to frequent infections and gum problems. Tobacco also decreases the vitamin C level in the body, which is needed to build healthy gum tissue.

Remedies: Try to stop smoking. Seek professional advice if you feel you can't succeed in quitting on your own. Vitamin supplements, especially vitamin C, are helpful in reducing the incidence of gum problems. See your dentist or dental hygienist frequently and create a good oral hygiene regimen.

3

Stress and Its Effect on Gum Disease

Stress upsets our normal bodily functions. How we react to outside stimuli affects both our physical and mental health. Stress causes a cycle, which perpetuates even more stress. When you encounter problems and experience anxiety and stress as a result, you may neglect yourself and then, in turn, your health can fail in many different ways. This can lead to more stress.

Everyone experiences stress on a daily basis. An important lesson to learn is not to immerse yourself in stress, but to work to separate yourself from it. You can achieve this by realizing stress is apart from who you are, and thereby mentally detaching yourself from the problem. Then try to work out the problem with the use of objective, intelligent choices.

The experience of stress, however, does affect your mouth and gums negatively. Your health will noticeably improve as you eliminate stress, or its negative impact, from your life.

Why Stress Is the Culprit

Stress is a result of an endocrine and hormonal imbalance. It affects the normal balance of your body and can lead to gum disease. The mouth mirrors many conditions of the body, especially those caused by stress. Headaches, which are usually stress-related, can restrict blood flow to the head. As a result of the loss of blood flow, you can get a headache. Chronic stress can lead to gum disease by reducing the strength of the immune system, which leads to growth of bacterial plaque. This bacterial plaque can invade the gum structure and lead to loose, inflamed tissue, as well as possible bone loss.

If you are stressed out and not paying much attention to your body's needs, you may be the victim of a poor diet, an important factor in gum disease. Most people who are under the influence of stress eat improperly. Your diet may consist of quick bites of food, sugar, or alcohol, and reduced intake of fluids. If you eat a high-sugar diet, you are certain to have a more acidic saliva, and probably will be a candidate for bacterial plaque. The bacterial plaque will irritate your gums and be a cause of gum disease. Alcohol, as discussed in the previous chapter, has a high sugar content and also diminishes the saliva flow, which is a cause of gum disease. If you drink less water and take in less fluid because of stress, you may notice your saliva thickening. This can cause plaque to attach quickly to the tooth's structure. Plaque feasts on the fragile gum tissue and eats away at the bone supporting the teeth.

Stress can also cause bad physical habits that can wreak havoc on your mouth. Have you ever been in the supermarket, waiting on line for what seems an eternity, and noticed that the person in front of you is overusing his jaws? You can tell by the facial musculature. Grinding and clenching of your teeth can loosen your teeth, and the pressure it produces can irritate the supporting gum tissue. In children, a loose baby tooth can cause the gum to get loose and swollen. Well, when you grind and clench your adult teeth, you are loosening them, and this can have the same effect as a loose baby tooth: it can cause loose, irritated gum tissue, which can result in gum disease.

Colds are also a direct effect of a weakened immune system. With colds and allergies affecting our immune system, the mouth can become a secondary target, with the resulting effect of gum disease.

However, *positive* stress can help our health and reduce anxiety. Stressful situations can lead us to challenge our spirit and sometimes leave us healthier. It's how we *react* to stress that is important. If you handle your problems well, you may achieve a healthier immune system.

All in all, however, I would suggest that you try to minimize the stress in your life, for it can play havoc not only on your gums but on other organs such as your heart. Although stress may not be considered a disease, it can be the aggravating factor for such conditions as allergies, arthritis, asthma, cancer, colitis, ulcers, heart disease, and various nerve conditions. These conditions can all have an effect on your gum tissue.

As mentioned earlier, stress may lead you away from good daily gum and tooth care. You may be preoccupied with your problems and so neglect your body. However, you can start to release your frustrations through positive manipulation of the gum tissue. Think about how good a gum massage feels. It can relax you. If you spend a minute or two in the morning with gum massage, you will relax your mouth and heal the gum tissue.

Using the Mind-Body-Spirit Connection to Eliminate the Effects of Stress

The mind-body-spirit connection to stress embraces the probability that stress can contribute to illness. In a positive state, the mind promotes better immune functioning for the body. Our will, or spirit, contributes to our well-being. Depression can lead to ill health and bad habits that can lead to disease. If your spirit is low, it can lower the immune system and bring on disease. Stress comes from lack of hope and leads to negative or ill health. Ill health can cause more stress. If you are under stress, use your mind to control your experience of stress.

While negative thoughts cause a lowering of the immune system and disease, positive thoughts can enhance the immune system. It is the spirit within us that needs to guide us positively. Use the mind-body-spirit connection to transform stress into positive energy. Life is a series of lessons to be learned, and once they are learned, their adversity can disappear. The mind-body-spirit connection can control our level of stress. If a problem exists and you do your daily cleaning routine, emphasizing your health first, it will help you put stress into proper perspective.

Feelings of hope and renewed optimism can promote better immune function for the body. Hope and optimism reduce fear and allow the body to move in a positive direction.

Stress and its connection to oral health are not addressed in textbooks or scientifically recorded. I have observed that many of my patients, however, when tired and stressed out, seem to have puffy and swollen gum tissue. After changing jobs or returning from vacations, these same patients suddenly have remarkably healthy tissue. Stress-related problems have been studied in dentistry, and the findings in many countries are that when there is less stress, there are fewer problems with teeth and gums.

Stress-Related Habits That Worsen Gum Disease

Bruxism

If you find that your jaws are tight when you awake, you may be clenching and grinding your teeth in your sleep. The grinding and clenching of teeth is a habit called bruxism, and it is caused by stress. Clenching is a continuous or periodic closing of the jaw under vertical pressure. Grinding is a rhythmic side-to-side movement or a forward-and-back movement. The teeth are under severe pressure when you clench and grind them. The constant moving of your teeth back and forth while grinding will loosen the teeth.

If you grind and clench your teeth, you may find yourself with a condition called temporomandibular joint disorder (TMJ). The temporomandibular joint is the hinge and socket that allow the mouth to open and close. The jaw can sometimes lock into position, limiting your mouth in opening and closing. Or you may hear clicking sounds, indicating that the TMJ is not working as smoothly as it should. Grinding or clenching your teeth inhibits the correct movement of this joint. Stretching the ligaments creates problems for the TMJ joint and can even affect your gum condition. It can inhibit your ability to do proper oral hygiene and can cause pain, leading to stress in your mouth and causing you to feel uncomfortable.

The amount of damage that you can do to your mouth correlates directly with the duration of the grinding-and-clenching habit. Bruxism will show as wear on your teeth. If you routinely grind your teeth in your sleep and clench daily, then you will probably cause serious damage to your teeth. Headaches may even be due to the grinding and clenching of your teeth, as they place excess stress on the ligaments and supportive tissues.

Breaking such a habit is hard because it is usually a secondary factor to major stress. It takes awareness, and a conscious willingness to change the behavior pattern, to stop the bad habit.

Remedies: If you are consciously aware that you are clenching, then use your tongue as a tool to inhibit the process and place it between your teeth. In the evenings before retiring, drink a glass of warm milk and relax. *Do not* go over your worries for the day as you prepare for slumber: think pleasant thoughts, especially before going into a dream state.

If your jaws are tight and you are in pain, you might want to try some isometric exercises. Isometric means *resistance.* Cup your hands under your chin and press upward while your mouth muscles push your chin down onto your hands. Do the same with the side of your jaw: press your jaw to one side while you press in with your cupped hands, one on either side of your jaw. Resistance in this area will strengthen the ligaments and lead the TMJ back to health. If you are getting headaches due to clenching and grinding, this will help to eliminate the pressure and allow the circulation of blood to the brain, thus eliminating the headaches.

If you are grinding and clenching your teeth in your sleep, you will have little control over the habit. A night guard or splint can be made to enable you to keep your teeth apart at night. If you feel that you can wear this comfortably, make an appointment with your dental professional to have one made. Your dentist will take an impression, make a mold, and send the mold to a lab to make you a customized night guard or splint. Night guards sold in drugstores over the counter will not fit properly, and can irritate the gum tissue. An ill-fitting night guard or tray can be the cause of gum disease.

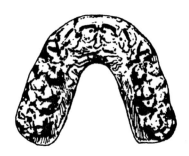

A night guard.

Cheek Biting

Chewing on the lining of your cheeks and biting your lips may be a nervous habit. This may lead to ulcers and irritation. Irritation of your cheeks will make it difficult for you to effectively perform oral hygiene, thus possibly leading to gum disease. Ulcers in your mouth can spread and irritate the gum tissue.

Remedies: Consciously try to stop this habit. Stress can cause us to hurt our body parts. Remind yourself of the good that is in your life, and that you can decrease your stress level and bad habits.

Instead of biting your cheek, place a rubber band on your wrist. Every time you are about to bite your cheek, snap the rubber band. After a while you will stop biting your cheek (and also will not have to snap the rubber band that is on your wrist!). The rubber band is more obvious, and your conscious mind will not allow the pain that is a consequence of this negative habit to continue.

Ice Chewing

Another bad habit caused by stress is chewing on ice. Ice can be very destructive and cause much harm to the teeth. It can wear down the surfaces of your teeth as well as irritate the gums because of the excess stress you are placing on your teeth with the ice. This all depends, of course, on the severity of the habit.

Remedies: Awareness of the damage that chewing on ice can do to your teeth and gums will help you to break the habit. Consciously remember this at the times you may want to chew on ice. Remove these thoughts and replace them with positive thoughts.

If you chew ice as a stress reliever, you might find that you will break many of your teeth. Such knowledge works to curb the habit. It causes you to be conscious that you can make the enamel thin with the habit of ice chewing, which will lead you to have sensitive teeth. And sensitive teeth can cause you pain. Pain and sensitivity will not allow you to enjoy good foods. If you need to release stress in this fashion, chew sugarless gum instead.

Gum Chewing

If stress is leading you to chew gum, choose sugarless gum. It is important to note that the chewing of gum is not always negative; it increases the saliva flow, which cleanses the teeth and adds moisture to gum tissue. If you constantly chew gum and find that your jaw is sore, you may be over-doing it. Chewing sugarless gum in moderation can be helpful, as it can reduce stress and lubricate the mouth.

Remedies: Chew in moderation. If you think you are relieving stress by chewing gum, then chances are you are probably overdoing it. Too much stress on the jaw is tiring and can cause the mouth to get irritated. Try to let go by working out instead—going for a walk or jog, biking, or swimming. If you find that you need an oral fix, then chew on carrot or celery sticks. Stress is removed by healthful foods. Do not allow yourself to enter the realm of negativity.

Gum chewing in excess can be a cause for muscle stress in your mouth. If you chew, chew sugarless gum, and do so in moderation.

Eating Sweets

Stress can cause us to act irrationally and can lead us to want to erase any negative feelings by eating sweets. It is known that chocolate can compensate for romance, and it affects the pituitary gland. What does it do to our teeth and fragile gum tissue? Try placing sweetened chocolate and other sweets on your skin. You will find they will irritate the skin. They will also irritate the oral cavity. Sugar turns to acid, and acid eats away at the soft and hard tissues of the oral cavity. Plaque and bacteria feed off the sugar and invade the support structures of your teeth.

Remedies: A conscious effort and a focused mind will help you to stop eating sweets at times of duress. Replace the belief that negative feelings are extinguished when you eat sweets, and instead eat foods that are good for you, like fruits such as apples, bananas, and strawberries, and vegetables such as broccoli, spinach, and dark green lettuce. I have recently tried to diet, and I find that when I am stressed out I tend to eat something that gives me instant gratification such as chocolate. I then realize I like some really good foods such as strawberries and watermelon. I use self-control and eat healthily and feel better. The existing balance of your energy system in your body will help you to reduce stress.

Do not keep sweets in the house. If you thrive on chocolate and sweets due to a high level of stress, remind yourself of the cycle into which it can lead you: weight gain, the lack of necessary vitamins, an acidic mouth produced by sugar intake and poor diet, and loose gum tissue. All this will create additional stress. Try to reduce, and not increase, your stress level, by exercising control; you will eliminate stress quicker. Sweet eaters are instant gratification seekers, but you can become an educated consumer. Think healthily and exercise your body. Drink more water and eat nutritious foods. This practice of healthy thinking will eliminate the need for sweets.

Vitamin Deficiency

Stressful behavior patterns can lead to vitamin deficiencies. When people are under stress, sucrose ingestion may lead to hypoglycemia, a condition directly related to stress. The National Institutes of Health reports that 87 percent of the population suffer from faulty carbohydrate metabolism. Eating improperly, which usually occurs when a person is under stress, can lead to lack of vitamins.

Remedies: Take vitamin supplements at times of stress. Magnesium and zinc, along with a multiple vitamin, can be very helpful.

If you find that you are not eating properly and are in need of vitamins, take supplemental vitamins in pill form. Vitamin supplements are easy to buy, and it is important when you are going through stressful times to supplement the body's needs. Vitamins build strong bone that supports your teeth and helps to generate gum tissue. Stress will throw the body off balance, and these vitamins are very important to feed both the teeth and gums. Also, exercising will help with circulation and help prevent the vitamin depletion in your body.

Nail Biting/Thumb Sucking

Thumb sucking and nail biting are habits related to stress. You may laugh, but many adults do habitually suck their thumbs.

These oral habits, which arise from stress, can cause gum disease. The nails beds are loaded with bacteria and when placed in the mouth can contribute to an environment rich in bacteria, thus irritating the gum tissue. Think about it: You touch things all day that are laden with bacteria and then you place your fingers in your mouth, chewing the nail off and leaving the bacteria to invade the soft tissues of your mouth. These stress-related habits can contribute to gum infection and may even contribute to gum abscesses. If you have a cut on your gum and then bite your nails, the bacteria that are introduced can lodge in the cut, causing an abscess.

Remedies: Have a professional manicure weekly. The cost and effort spent to beautify your nails will help you to eliminate the bad habit of putting your hands in your mouth.

A beautiful manicure will cost you money but it will eliminate the bacteria from spreading into your mouth due to nail biting, and may even help reduce your stress level.

Lemon Sucking

Sucking lemons is another habit caused by stress. Do you know how acidic lemons are? Acid is *not* a friend to the soft tissues of your mouth. It can dry and irritate the soft tissue. I have heard about people sucking on lemons as a relaxant! People do different, quirky things when they are stressed. Most of the time, these things are deleterious to the mouth and other parts of the body.

Remedies: Herbal candies can be a good replacement. The need to have an oral fixation is better replaced with herbal components.

Habitual lemon sucking can cause much damage to the supporting structures of your teeth. If you find that you are sucking on lemons excessively due to stress, consciously make an effort to stop, and intellectually understand that this habit can damage your teeth and gums. Think of the sour taste in your mouth. Does this really make you feel good? Exercise your good sense and replace the acidic lemon with some cooling fruits and vegetables. Cucumbers are very cooling to the gum tissue, so place them on the gums instead. Cooling fruits and vegetables will allow the gums to heal in times of stress.

Toothbrush Abrasion and Stress

Many people use their toothbrush too harshly and take out their frustrations by brushing too hard, causing toothbrush

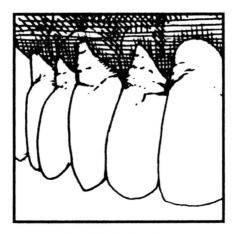

Toothbrush abrasion.

abrasion. This can end up ridging the enamel of your teeth. Enamel is a veneer that can be ridged by a hard brush or heavy-handed brushing. The ridge line that many professionals see is close to the gum line. This ridge can become a holding place for food and plaque to attach to. This area, if grooved deeply, will collect bacterial plaque that can be a cause of gum disease. If toothbrush abrasion causes you pain and sensitivity, then you may not be working effectively at removing the plaque and tartar from your gums.

Remedies: Use a soft brush and angle it with a massage approach at the gum line. Stressful times lead us to beat up on the soft tissue of the mouth, so consciously become aware of how hard you are working your mouth. Examine your teeth, and if any ridges are appearing on the tooth line, then stop any harsh strokes. Nurture yourself.

Toothbrush abrasion is a common result of anger and stress. Many people brush harshly at the gum line and cause their gums to recede (shrink), leaving them "long in the tooth." Consciously massage the gums and let your hands relax before you approach your mouth with the brush. Use rhythm, much as you would if you were exercising your body at the gym.

Alcohol Use

Drinking alcohol to reduce stress can lead to more stress. Stress has to be brought to a level of awareness and dealt with. Alcohol reduces the ability to deal with problems, thus creating a severe problem in itself. It also causes bad gums and diminishes saliva flow, thus drying out the gum tissue. This dried gum tissue will become sore and loose and can be a factor in the onset of gum disease.

Remedies: If you are deeply involved in alcohol use, seek professional or group help. Motivate yourself to act by knowing that alcohol depletes all the vitamins in your system and eats away at your tooth structures.

If you are stressed and are turning to alcohol, try to problem-solve instead, and think clearly. Throw away the alcohol and face your problems. Lead yourself into an environment that is healthier and cleaner. Try yoga, or another form of exercise, and breathe deeply and slowly.

Tobacco Smoking

Another stress-related habit is smoking. Smoking can destroy your health because cigarettes contain thousands of toxins. Smoking is immunosuppressive, and it may take over three months to reverse the damage it causes. The use of tobacco products puts you at a high risk of periodontal disease. Tobacco smoking has been associated with acute necrotizing ulcerative gingivitis (ANUG), a severe form of gingivitis. Nicotine use can reduce antibody production, alter T-cell ratios, and reduce the mineral content in the bones. All of these reactions to nicotine can affect your gums. When you look at people who smoke, notice their facial skin. Just as smoking dries the tissue of the face, leaving the skin lined and wrinkled, it also dries out the gums.

Remedies: Try SmokeEnders or hypnosis, or just go cold turkey. Throw away your demons. If this doesn't work, seek professional help. Go to your doctor and get a prescription for the nicotine patch. If you are an habitual smoker and find that during stressful times you smoke more, consciously make an effort to reduce your smoking. You may think you are getting relief from smoking, but it is actually increasing your stress level. Fight the bad habits and challenge yourself to achieve good health by problem-solving instead.

Knowing that stress is one of the problems that can cause illness and gum disease is very important. But just knowing is not enough; it takes willpower and self-control to eliminate the stressful habits. In times of excessive stress, think of your body as a machine; do not overwork the physical machine with bad habits and negative thoughts. Let problem-solving lead you in the right direction. Thought processes create energy, which can elevate or lower your immune system. Positive problem-solving will lead to better health and help you eliminate stresses leading to gum disease. And, most important, *throw away your tobacco.* I am not a psychologist, but I have noticed that most people who smoke have control issues. What is in control here, the tobacco? Are you letting the tobacco lead you to ill health? Exercise your intelligence and logically understand your need for this habitual life-reducing substance. Then reduce the need to have addictions that do not promote your health.

In this chapter I focused on some of the most common bad habits that may be the cause of gum disease. If you catch the problems early, you will have less trouble reducing or breaking them. Stress can be a negative energy force that enters our life and invades our bodies. Don't let it impact your life, or your body, in a negative way.

PART II

HEALING MODALITIES AND TOTAL BODY CARE

In this part, you will be introduced to a line of natural herbal products and the old-fashioned baking soda products that can do wonders for your mouth. You will also discover that the mouth is connected to meridians that connect to our body's organs. Everything connects to something else. Gum disease is related to the immune system, and the entire body should be considered.

4

Handling Pain and Fear

Pain can be considered a major cause of dental problems and gum disease. If you are afraid of pain and associate visits to the dentist or hygienist with a painful experience, you probably will not be visiting your dentist office often enough. Missing your regular check-ups will lead you to neglect your teeth and gums, and can result in the onset of gum disease.

Pain is an unpleasant sensory and emotional experience. It is caused by the stimulation of sensory nerve endings, which the mouth has an abundance of. Every person perceives pain differently. Social, cultural, and ethnic differences affect how different people react to pain. Pain can be an intense experience, and even if there is no actual physical reason for it, the person feels the pain as if it is real.

Is pain always present when there is gum disease? No, not always. Pain is not present when your gums are inflamed, bleeding, or swollen. However, any problems that cause pain in the mouth may also contribute to gum disease. For example, disease can become a secondary problem if you have pericoronitis (swollen gums around the wisdom teeth). The tissue can become inflamed as a result of the crowding, and bacteria lodged in one area can spread to adjacent tissue. An abscess—an area in the gum filled with pus—may be painful. If your mouth is sore because of temporomandibular disorder, then the surrounding tissue can also be affected, leaving you with raw, swollen gums. Neuralgia in the facial area may leave you uncomfortable and may induce you not to practice proper dental hygiene home care. A burning tongue may leave you irritated and discourage you from nurturing your oral cavity, resulting in gum disease. So any discomfort in your mouth may lead you to gum disease.

Mouth Conditions That Can Cause Pain

Let us look more closely at the common conditions of the mouth that can cause pain.

Somatic Pain Disorder

This condition stems from local (oral/periodontal) tissue injury, and shows up as inflammation and local tooth problems, such as decay.

For example, you go to the hygienist for a thorough cleaning and now your gums feel raw and swollen. After leaving the office, you are having a sensation of pain. (Does this sensation make you feel that you want to return for another cleaning? No!)

My patients don't experience this pain sensation, because after a gum treatment I massage the tissue therapeutically with herbal toothpaste and clove oil or oreganol on a toothbrush. During a cleansing treatment, I dip the instrument into the oil to lubricate and numb the tissue. Most patients feel soothed and nurtured after a treatment, and end up asking to come back.

Remedies: Have clove oil on hand for emergencies. If you feel pain on a particular tooth, dab a Q-tip into the clove oil and swab the oil onto the tooth surface. This will remove the painful sensation. However, if you see a dentist or hygienist regularly, a painful situation like this will occur much less frequently. Prevention can keep painful situations from occurring.

Abscess

Another cause of mouth pain may be an abscess, which is a localized infection of either the gums or a decayed tooth. A raw or abscessed gum can cause pain, and may even feel like a toothache or a nerve dying. The painful sensation will probably come on when you are drinking or eating cold food. Look in the mirror and see if you can locate the source of the pain.

Remedies: If your gum is raw and swollen and you see a bump on the gum that might be an abscess, rinse with warm sea salt water to draw the infection out. To reduce swelling, steep a tea bag in boiling water. Remove the tea bag from the water, let it cool, and place the bag on the source of the pain. The tannic acid in the tea bag will reduce the swelling and calm the irritation until you see your dentist or hygienist.

Pericoronitis

This condition is due to the impaction, or crowding, of wisdom teeth. Wisdom teeth are found in the back of your mouth. Because of crowding, the area around the wisdom tooth may be hard to reach for cleaning purposes. The gum that surrounds this area then can get swollen and loose.

Remedies: Use an oral irrigator with peroxide (see chapter 5). Also, seek the advice of a dentist or an hygienist. To eliminate swelling, pour boiling water over a tea bag. Remove the bag from the water and let it cool. Then place the tea bag over the wisdom teeth that are causing you problems and bite down. You may get a sense of relief.

Trigeminal Neuralgia

There are only three to five cases per year per 100,000 people with this condition, and it is more common in those over fifty years of age. In this condition, you may think that you have a toothache when the pain isn't really related to a tooth. Still, to rule out the possibility that it's not a toothache, seek professional dental advice. A symptom of this condition may be that you have pain-free intervals—the pain comes and goes without reason. If a dental condition or a tooth problem causes your pain, you will have a continuous aching, throbbing pain. Any stimulation worsens the pain. With trigeminal neuralgia, you feel only intermittent, brief, electric shock–like pain. A light touch will trigger the pain, which is part of trigeminal neuralgia. This condition is frequently misdiagnosed by dentists.

Remedies: Seek professional advice and have your dentist or physician diagnose the problem. You should be treated for this condition professionally.

Phantom Pain (Atypical Facial Pain)

Phantom pain is a persistent pain in the teeth, face, or alveolar process (bone) following a root canal therapy, an apicoectomy (surgical removal of an infection or cyst), or a tooth extraction. It may be a deep, dull ache with periodic sharp attacks. Three to six percent of those who undergo a root canal therapy have a phantom pain sensation in the area of the treated tooth. Phantom pain also is often experienced in people who have lost limbs; they can still "feel" the presence of the limb and pain that does not diminish in that area.

Remedies: Check with your dentist, who will try to determine the source of your pain and proceed with the professional treatment of choice.

Burning Mouth

Burning mouth is an intraoral chronic pain disorder that is usually without associated mucosal or oral signs. You may feel a burning sensation on your tongue, and stinging and itching in the front and back regions of your tongue. It can be caused by a geographic tongue (inflammation sporadically mapped out on your tongue) or an infection such as candidiasis. Or you may have a contact allergy from wearing dentures.

Other causes may be a nervous condition, such as the biting of one's tongue or other tongue habits, or an allergic reaction to medications being taken. A person can have burning of the tongue or surrounding areas if he or she is anemic; with this condition there is a reddened area on the tongue called glossitis. This condition is either continuous or intermittent, and typically worsens as the day progresses. It is relieved temporarily by eating and drinking. It is estimated that 8 percent of males and 6 percent of females suffer from this condition.

Remedies: Seek a physician's advice rather than that of a dentist.

Temporomandibular Disorder (TMD)

Still another painful condition is related to temporomandibular disorder. The temporomandibular joint (TMJ) is the joint by the ear that allows the mouth to open and close. This joint can become arthritic, much as any joint in your body can, and can cause you pain.

Usually people complain about arthritis in their knees or in the joints of their fingers. But every joint is composed of synovial fluid and ligament attachment, and thus is subject to arthritis. A dental professional may be called on to locate and manage the complaints that occur around the TMJ.

Remedies: The treatment of choice by a dentist probably would be a night guard. This will not cure the condition, however, if the joint itself is arthritic, only ease the discomfort.

To relieve pain immediately, use warm compresses on the outside of the joint.

Mouth Ulcers

Often found in adults and teenagers, ulcers are indicative of a run-down physical condition. These open sores in the mouth can also occur after antibiotic therapy and during recovery from influenza. When the body's immune system experiences much stress, the normal ecology of the mouth is compromised. Ulcers can be very painful, especially when one is eating and drinking.

Remedies: A mouthwash made with red sage leaves or echinacea by Bioforce will usually reduce the pain.

Children and Pain in Dentistry

Luckily, there is usually little pain experienced by children who have gum problems. The child first realizes something is wrong when he or she sees blood on his or her toothbrush, which is usually due to sore tissue. Still, here are the conditions that can cause pain.

Abscess

This is a localized infection of the gums or a decayed tooth. The pressure of the pus and diseased gum may cause discomfort and some pain in children as much as in adults.

Remedies: Seek professional advice. Use of a tea bag can be helpful—after steeping a tea bag in hot water, let it cool and place it on the abscess. The tannic acid will draw the infection out. A rinse with warm sea salt water can also be helpful. Have your child swish the rinse around his or her mouth. If the problem persists after a dental cleaning, then seek the advice of a physician. Make sure your child develops good oral hygiene habits.

Tooth Decay

From treating many children in dental hygiene, I've noticed that children seem to experience less pain with tooth decay than adults do. I have worked on many children with rampant decay, and their parents, as well as the children themselves, were unaware of any problems. Most decay is noticed only when the teeth are darkened with severe amounts of decay.

Remedies: For temporary relief, apply clove oil. Then make an appointment to have the decay removed and a filling or proper tooth restoration applied.

Teething

The earliest and most common pain in a child is related to teething, when the baby tooth pushes up and breaks through the gum. The symptoms of teething are excessive saliva in the mouth, sometimes a fever, crankiness, and sleeplessness.

In response to teething pain, a child will grab almost anything and start chewing on it. As the pressure of the new teeth erupting causes discomfort, the counterpressure created by using objects or fingers will alleviate some of the pain.

Teething occurs in all children, and the immune system sometimes becomes involved during the creation of excess mucus in children. The child may run a temperature. Do not become alarmed! Fever is a common side effect of teething in a child.

Remedies: Pressure from the eruption of a tooth will cause the fibers in the gums to give a painful sensation to your child. Natural remedies can help reduce the pain. Clove oil is the most effective natural numbing solution. Spread it over the area that is causing discomfort with a cotton swab. Use teething rings that have been kept cold in the refrigerator. The cold on the gums and the clove oil will aid in numbing the painful gums. If a fever persists, seek a physician's advice.

Eliminating Fear

What keeps people away from dental treatment? It is usually fear and anxiety. An unpleasant past experience, or hearing about negative experiences from other people, is probably a major cause of dental disease and gum disease.

Children who have had a negative experience in a dental office may harbor negative thoughts for a lifetime. As children often do not understand what is happening to them in the dental chair, they feel out of control. This lack of control can play havoc with the mind. Negative experiences during childhood then become magnified over time and are hard to forget, creating an atmosphere of fear every time an adult thinks about going to the dentist or hygienist.

If you are an adult who carries fears from childhood, sometimes eliminating your fear can be as easy as remembering (and perhaps discussing!) the original painful incident from your childhood. Also, express your concerns to your dental professional. The right dental professional will be empathetic and understanding. And most dental offices are equipped to reduce the pain experience. Discuss with your dentist or hygienist the various methods that might work for you during treatment to alleviate pain, and remember that the less pain you experience, the better it is for you *and* your professional. If you tense up with fear, it becomes more difficult for your professional to do the best job possible. So it is in everyone's best interests that you are less fearful and do not have to contend with pain.

It is important to educate children in dental care. There is a child in all of us, and if a strong foundation has been built first, we can become healthy and fearless adults. If as a child we were unexpectedly hurt in the dental chair—we didn't expect to have a needle or a drill—then as adults we remain fearful of the dentist.

So educate your children in dental care, and explain to them why they must fix their teeth. It is important to have your child understand the need to see a dentist and dental hygienist. It would be advantageous to have your child visit the dentist with you and let him or her look at the equipment. Ask the dentist if you can have a half-hour consultation to make your child more comfortable in the dental chair. This visit would be to familiarize your child with dental equipment, and when it becomes his or her time to be a patient, he or she will have gained knowledge. Any fear will be eliminated or lessened.

I remember, as a child, pinching my hand to remove the sensation of pain from the actual area being worked on. It works! It makes your mind concentrate on a sharper pain that *you* are in control of. Try it.

Also, try to eliminate fear with logic. Think of the most traumatic pain you have ever undergone. The pain sensation that you experienced may well have disappeared in a few minutes and was not long-lasting. Chronic pain that gnaws at you daily can be considered stressful pain.

Reducing Our Stress Level

There is a direct link between mental and emotional distress and the body's physical health. Mental and emotional stress—brought about by things like the pain and fear we've been discussing—can weaken the immune system, allowing disease to take hold in the body. A lowered immune system response is one of the major factors in the onset of gum disease.

Pain and the stress that causes fear are related to the development of gum disease. To help eliminate the cause and onset of gum disease, and to promote its reversal, we must work to reduce the level of stress we are experiencing physically, mentally, and emotionally.

The following treatments and techniques will help you to reverse gum disease naturally by reducing your stress and pain levels that are caused by dental fears and related problems.

Yoga

Yoga comes from the word "yoke"; in Sanskrit the word means "union." Our mouth is connected to our body, and we must heal our mouth much the same as we would heal our body. A positive mind is a mind that can heal.

The most widely known yoga practice is asana, often known as hatha yoga. Asana means "ease" in Sanskrit and includes a variety of physical postures that create changes in the body. Although yoga emphasizes little movement, the mind is involved with each asana, and thus a mind-body-spirit connection is made. The connection of the breath and the mind is a basic principle of yoga. If the mind is balanced and focused, the breath will be focused and still.

Pranayama focuses on the regulation of the breath. The prana exercises are taught to remove energy blockages and prevent illnesses.

If the mind is restless and agitated, the breathing system will become the same. Doing prana exercises induces deep breathing and leads to relaxation of the body and its organs. The added oxygen will help heal the organs of the body and clear the mind. Prana has also been shown to help digestion, improve cardiac function, and strengthen the immune system. If the immune system is enhanced, then all conditions of weakness in the body can be reversed.

Meditation, also used in yoga, is a state of focus that heightens your awareness, relaxing you into peace and harmony. Using both yoga and meditation will enhance your immune system, thus alleviating weakness.

Children, too, can benefit from the study of yoga. They can start at a young age to learn the patterns and postures of yoga for preventive measures to build their immune system. Children love movement, and they are usually more flexible than adults.

If you wish to get a feel for hatha yoga, find a comfortable place in a dimly lit room. You can have some incense burning if you wish. For more information please seek out a class or videotape. Try these three positions:

1. *Child's posture:* Sit in a kneeling position on the floor and let your arms hang by your side. Relax your arms

and rest your hands by your side. The back should be curved. In this position, the hands and body are completely relaxed. Hold the posture for about five minutes.

2. *Shoulder stand:* Lie on your back with your legs apart. Raise both legs until they are perpendicular to the floor, lifting the hips toward the ceiling. Press the breastbone toward the chin.

3. *Half fish:* Sit with your head, neck, and trunk straight. Your legs should be pressed together and extended in front of your body. Lean back and place your elbows and forearms on the floor in line with your body and legs. Arch your back, expanding your chest and stretching your neck backward until you can place the crown of your head on the floor. Now breathe evenly for twenty seconds.

Exercise

When you exercise regularly, you begin to improve the condition of your heart and lungs. Exercise releases toxins from your body and improves your stamina. It increases your blood circulation and your joint mobility. It also alleviates premenstrual stress or stress experienced during menopause. It strengthens your bones by increasing their mineral content; therefore, it helps in reducing osteoporosis and enhances the bone level in your mouth. The bone in your mouth surrounds the roots of your teeth, giving the teeth support. So if you exercise regularly, you will reduce gum disease and increase the circulation that is needed for healthy gum tissue.

Here are some suggestions for ways in which to exercise. Play golf, which enhances the cardiovascular system. Tennis generates good muscular action and circulation. Walking is less jarring to the joints than jogging or running and also helps the cardiovascular system and circulation. Swimming will enhance the mobility of your joints and increase your circulation and cardiovascular system. Getting twenty to thirty minutes of aerobic exercise three to five times a week can be beneficial to your health and enhance your immune system.

Exercise is also a natural antidepressant. Physiological changes in the body and brain that result from exercise can elevate your mental state. When you exercise, you increase your body's temperature by two or three degrees, which is relaxing. Endorphins also are released, which enhance the immune system and give us a sense of elation and well-being. Many runners have described a feeling of being "high" when running or jogging.

Still, motivating yourself to exercise regularly may be as difficult as motivating yourself to do a daily oral hygiene regimen. It might be more difficult if you feel that you are lacking energy. If you do exercise that you enjoy, you may be more motivated than if you hate the exercise you plan for yourself. So whichever activity you choose, enjoy it. Using your energy in a positive way will make you feel better and look younger.

Dance Movements for Stress Reduction

Dance and movement are recognized by many as a stimulant for the immune system. It is a therapy used to release stress and reduce pain. Personality is connected to movement, and the release of personal expression through dance therapy also helps reduce depression. I advise dancing in group sessions, starting with warm-up sessions.

Rhythm, which one develops through dance, does play a factor in the treatment of the mouth. You can massage with your brush, floss, and other oral products using a fashionable dance rhythm. The tedium of oral care will be reduced, and you will send healing energy through this rhythm from your hands to your mouth.

Biofeedback

Machines and instruments are used in biofeedback to help you learn to self-regulate your body functions, and to control your blood pressure and heart rate. Electronic beeps and flashes provide information about the body's changes, and by responding to these signals, you can learn (with the help of a practitioner) how to regulate your body's response. If you have anxiety about going to the dentist, you may learn to regulate your blood pressure and heart rate with biofeedback procedures, which will be very helpful in controlling anxiety about dental treatment. Stress and pain relief can be altered with biofeedback methods.

Different kinds of biofeedback methods are available. There are devices that show you changes in your skin temperature. A GSR device measures the skin's electrical conductivity by the amount of sweat produced under stress. EMGs are visual signals that indicate muscle tension. If you are in a state of relaxation, your sweat glands will have low activity, and high levels of alpha waves in the brain will indicate a slow, even heart rate. You can begin to train yourself to regulate your body's organs through the use of such equipment. Many people who have undergone biofeedback therapy have achieved control over fears, stress, and pain.

Diet

I discuss various foods throughout this book to help keep your body healthy. The most successful diet in terms of stress reduction is to *stay away from sugar.* If you were to care for a car or any other machine you wish to run smoothly, then you would give it quality fuel. The same holds true for your body: to have energy and be healthy, you must eat foods that fuel you with optimum nutrition. Also avoid junk food because such snack foods contain chemicals. This does not mean that when you are depressed you should eat sugar and carbohydrates. Foods loaded with sugar and carbohydrates will harm your body and eat away at your teeth and gums. These chemicals act as toxins in our cells and cause illness and disease.

Foods that can contribute to a bad mood include chocolate, which contains chemicals and stimulants, and coffee, which can also stimulate us. High-protein foods such as meat and eggs can help lift our spirits. Foods that contain starch and sugar-rich carbohydrates, such as potatoes and bread, increase blood sugar and can raise serotonin levels in the body. The serotonin levels in the body are usually low when a person is in a depression.

Ignore any desire for bad foods and try to exercise good eating habits, even if you are not in a positive frame of mind. Eating well and using self-control work toward elevating your spirits. They will also increase the well-being of your body.

Aromatherapy

Aromatherapy uses the medicinal properties found in the essential oils of plants to affect mood. Essential oils from herbal plants infused into oils (olive oil, for example) are either absorbed through the skin or inhaled. So either use them in oil that is rubbed into the skin or breathe them in through a diffuser.

The use of tea tree oil and lavender on top of toothpaste can relax you and soothe your gum tissue. They have a pleasant aroma, and are best to use before bedtime. Chamomile is also an excellent relaxant and can be used as an extract on top of toothpaste.

Here are some specifics about the calming oils:

- *Lavender:* Used for burns and small injuries. Its high ester content can give off a calming sensation to the brain.
- *Chamomile:* Calms an upset mind and can reduce mental and physical stress.
- *Mandarin:* Used as an oil, it can release anxiety.
- *Clary sage:* Used as a sedative.
- *Sandalwood:* Used as a sedative.

Any of these calming essences can be placed in a bath and used to calm and relax you. Add six drops to a warm bath and relax for ten to twenty minutes.

Acupuncture

Acupuncture can alleviate pain and enhance the immune system in response to a vital flow of life energy throughout the body. It can alter the perception of pain by intervening with neurotransmitters to the brain. Acupuncture stimulates the release of endorphins, the body's natural painkilling chemicals.

How does acupuncture work? There are twelve major pathways, or meridians, each linked to a specific organ, and there are over a thousand acupoints (meridian points). When needles are placed at these points, they stimulate the flow of *chi* (heart-released energy) in the body and remove blockages.

Massage Therapies

Massage therapy is effective in healing the whole body. Here are some different kinds of massage.

Reflexology

Foot massage. According to practitioners, when there is an imbalance in the body, granular crystalline substances are deposited on the reflex point. Can this correlation occur with the mouth? Can the blockage of the meridians in the mouth cause calcium deposits such as tartar? No research supports this theory at the present time, but it is possible.

In reflexology massage, pressure is placed on the meridians that run through the feet. Reflexology reduces stress and tension by increasing the blood flow that supplies the body. Much the same as acupuncture, reflexology removes the blocks that inhibit energy flow in the body.

Swedish Massage

Emotions can cause muscle tension and trap energy. This form of massage releases energy-bound muscles, reducing tension and relaxing the mind. This form of a massage can even put you into a sleep state.

Shiatsu Massage

This Eastern technique includes acupressure and aims to balance the energy of the body. The acupressure points are worked, and because of muscle relaxation, the mind also relaxes.

Aromatherapy Facial Massage

In this kind of massage, the practitioner will cleanse the skin and then follow with circular strokes with scented oils or creams. This is useful with the jaw muscles, which are often tense.

Qi-gong

This energy-based therapy can help the mind, body, and spirit in people of all ages. Qi-gong is the learning of breathing techniques and movements that stimulate the life force within the body. Stretching in front of the body can enhance lung capacity. Certain exercises will help you to recognize the *chi* energy within your body. Like acupuncture, qi-gong activates the electrical currents that flow within the pathways of the body and breaks down the energy blocks of the body.

Qi-gong can initiate a relaxing response, which decreases the sympathetic functions of the autonomic nervous system and frees the mind from distraction. This then increases blood flow to the capillaries and optimizes the delivery of oxygen to the tissue.

You can activate the *chi* in your body with a therapeutic gum massage that can also activate the immune system.

Qi-gong coordinates the left and right brain hemispheres, promoting deeper sleep, reduced anxiety, and mental clarity. It diminishes pain.

A simple way to get a sense of the *chi* in your body is to rub your hands together. After producing heat in your hands, place your hand over an organ. This will increase the *chi*. If you are interested in increasing the *chi* in the area of the mouth, then rub your hands together, producing heat, and place your hands over the region of the gums in your mouth. Feel your internal *chi* energy. See a practitioner of qi-gong for more specific information.

Tai Chi Ch'uan

This is a martial art form that uses breathing techniques with slow, graceful movements to improve the flow of *chi,* or life force, so that the mood is calmed. It is a meditation in motion performed by millions of Chinese people every day. There are 24 movements in the short version, and they can be performed in five to ten minutes. In the long version, there are 108 movements, which takes twenty to forty minutes to perform.

Visualization

By imagining positive images, you can overcome problems and heal yourself. Negative attitudes—including fear, pain, and stress—also can be changed with visualization.

I use imagery when I am in a situation that can be a painful experience. For example, when I go to the dentist to have a tooth drilled or even a root canal, instead of getting anesthesia I simply use my imagination and remove my mind from my body. This takes total concentration and meditation, but when I do so I am removed from any pain. I have surprised many practitioners with my abilities.

Hypnotherapy

Hypnosis is an artificially induced state characterized by a heightened receptivity to suggestion. This is achieved by relaxing the body and then shifting the mind to an object away from the body. If you reach a deep state of hypnosis, then a posthypnotic suggestion can be carried out. The deeper state of hypnosis can alter addictions by power of suggestion.

Hypnotherapy is very effective in treating stress and mental health problems such as fears and phobias, and even depression. It is used in psychology to remove fears and address problems. It can help a person stop smoking and overcome other harmful addictions. In dentistry, hypnotherapy is used with excellent results. It is known that hypnosis can control the circulatory system and enhance the healing process as well.

5

Working with Holistic Products for the Natural Reversal of Gum Disease

We've come a long way from the standard brush-and-floss routine. We have many alternative home dental care products that reach into every groove and crevice around the teeth and under the gum. If you have been told to brush and floss and are frustrated because you are not doing it properly, don't fear: there are alternatives to flossing. There have been new developments in hygiene and new products introduced. For example, there is now a proliferation of holistic products made from natural sources such as flowers and plants. It is important to use natural products for the body to heal with the least amount of toxicity. Read on, and you will see the advantages to using natural products for reversing gum disease as you learn how to properly clean your teeth and gums.

Why Is It Better to Use Natural Products?

The wide variety of products on the market can be confusing, but if you review the ingredients and select the most natural products, you will have positive results. The natural products I recommend, which can be purchased from many health food stores, offer the assurance that they contain:

- *No detergents:* Sodium lauryl sulfate (SLS) is a foaming agent that is found in most hair shampoos and is a highly allergenic component in many toothpastes. It is not needed for the health of your teeth and gums, and can cause irritation to the gums. The result might be gingivitis (inflammation of the gum).
- *No synthetic preservatives:* This lack of synthetic preservatives in toothpaste and mouthwash offers the tissue the purest form of healing allowed.
- *No saccharine or sugar:* Saccharine and sugar are not conducive to the health of gum tissue.
- *No artificial coloring:* Artificial coloring can irritate the gums and is only used to make a product attractive to the eye. Today, with everyone being so health conscious, it is no longer popular or advisable to add dye to a product.
- *No chemical whiteners:* These can irritate gum tissue and can be too abrasive to the teeth.
- *All natural ingredients:* The best products contain 100 percent natural ingredients.

Natural Products for Reversing Gum Disease

Flossing Products

At their healthiest, the interdental (in-between) areas of our teeth have an angle and a deeper pocket. Floss is an important tool to remove plaque and food debris in these areas. In my years of practicing dental hygiene, I have noticed that people do not floss correctly, and this causes more problems. A result of improper flossing is a cut on the gum tissue. Or, if people snap the floss, they cut the gum tissue and inflame the area. So do not snap the floss.

It is important to get in between the teeth and floss in a natural way. Products such as floss infused with natural herbs are easily obtained in health food stores. While floss is a treated string, if it contains natural herbs, it can assist in directing the herbal ingredients into the space between the teeth. Natural ingredients directed into areas that collect food and bacteria can assist in reversing gum disease naturally. So make sure you wrap the floss around the tooth under the gum.

To floss properly here is what you should do: Take approximately six to eight inches of flossing material from the container and wrap the floss (string) around your fingers comfortably, not too tight. Then gently wrap the tooth in a "C" shape. Remember, you're not just removing the food particles, but what you are doing is breaking loose plaque pedicles. Plaque attaches to the tooth and calcifies into tartar. So gently move the six to eight inches of the floss under the gum line and around the tooth. Proceed to the next tooth and apply the same procedure, remembering to wrap the floss around the tooth in a "C" shape.

Mouthwash

Herbal Mouthwash

The mouthwash used in my office is Bioforce Echinacea, an herbal mouthwash. It is a natural holistic composition of herbs that contains echinacea. Echinacea has been found to be a good wound healer for the oral cavity. I use it during gum cleansing. The mouth needs to be healed and soothed from time to time, and echinacea is soothing to the gums and can be used for prevention of soreness. It can help reduce fungus in your oral cavity, a cause of gum disease. I tell my patients to alternate it with water in an oral irrigator. It helps to moisturize and soothe the gum tissue while the action of the irrigator is at work. The mouth constantly needs to balance the pH level. Stress and spices added to foods alter the pH of the mouth. To stimulate the gums, put a drop of mouthwash on your toothbrush and massage the tissue. Other natural mouthwashes on the market are fortified with goldenseal, another herbal extract.

CoQ_{10} Mouthwash

There are many natural mouthwashes, and most of them can be found in health food stores. Some contain baking soda or coenzyme Q_{10}. Research shows that the use of CoQ_{10} can reduce gum disease. You can buy this product in capsules. Open a capsule and then apply the material on top of your toothpaste, or drop the powder into a liquid to make a rinse.

Rose Mouthwash

Red roses are more potent than any other colored rose (white, yellow, pink, violet, etc.). Rose petals have a large amount of vitamin C and will strengthen the gum tissue. If you have any red roses in your garden, gather up some of the petals that have fallen off the rose. Put the petals in a bowl and pour boiling water over them. Once the water has turned a deep rose color, you can use it for a mouthwash. You can also buy rose tea and prepare the tea as a mouth rinse.

Burdock Root

Burdock root can destroy a number of microorganisms that are responsible for gum disease. Prepare a concoction with one teaspoon of the root simmered in a cupful of water for fifteen minutes. Use it as a mouthwash, swishing it inside your mouth and holding it there for a few minutes at a time.

Natural Mouthwashes versus Commercial Brands

Sir Joseph Lister, who discovered the medical benefits of antiseptics, invented Listerine in 1879. Listerine originally was used as an antiseptic for cuts, scrapes, insect bites, and dandruff. You can find these same claims on the bottle today. In 1921 the company found another use for the product—thus the slogan, "Remember, nothing exceeds halitosis as a social offense. Nothing exceeds Listerine as a remedy." Due to the social connotation of bad breath and the smart advertising of Listerine, product sales increased. Despite its medicinal taste, this mouthwash still holds its own in sales. Today the company has colored the product with dye and has artificial ingredients in its composition. Rinses with dyes only mask breath odor. It is better to work on the real causes and help eliminate them. The mouth is always filled with bacteria, and when you are ill or eat certain foods the bacteria in your mouth multiply. Listerine may kill certain bacteria and at the same time may harm your delicate tissue with the chemicals and dyes in the product. The mouth should be treated like the skin on your face, and a gentle daily herbal rinse is preferred.

One cause of halitosis is the anaerobic bacteria that lie under the gum and also cause gum disease. Using peroxide in an oral irrigator can help eliminate the anaerobic bacteria under the gum. Peroxide is oxygen water, and oxygen is needed under the gum. However, if used as a mouthwash, it is not as effective. You must take precautions too with using peroxide as a mouthwash; it can be very caustic to the gum tissue over a long period of time (ten to twenty years of daily use). Alternate peroxide with an herbal mouthwash and sea salt, using them in a water pick.

Toothpaste

Do toothpastes feed tooth enamel and gum tissue, or do they just taste good to motivate patients to brush? Toothpaste manufacturers often advertise their toothpaste as either cosmetic or therapeutic. However, I have examined the ingredients in most of the big commercial-brand toothpastes. My findings were that most products contained the same ingredients but were just packaged differently.

Sweetened oral hygiene products will become less popular as people get the message, "Don't eat sweets."

Also, on the packaging for most toothpaste there is a phone number for poison control written on the tube of toothpaste. Few people take this message seriously. If the companies are writing this on their tubes of toothpaste, then they must have a *real* reason for doing so. I would rather use a good-quality natural herbal toothpaste that does not need to have this warning.

Natural Toothpaste

Echinacea Toothpaste

Used for dental health and gum care, this toothpaste not only cleans your teeth without being abrasive, but also feeds your gum tissue. Echinacea is extracted from several species of plants commonly called purple coneflower. Dr. Gerhard Madaus was the researcher who imported echinacea seeds from North America to Europe and scientifically studied them and found that they had immunostimulating properties. Echinacea is known to help heal surface wounds. It also helps heal gums that are sore and irritated.

Rosemary Toothpaste

Rosemary is found in the evergreen shrub and helps stimulate the blood flow in gum tissue. I find it works well on people who have receding (shrinking) gums. It activates the metabolism of the outer layer of gum tissue and improves cell regeneration. It is important to remember that tissue regenerates itself, so if you have receding gums, with the proper care and hygiene this tissue will grow back and become healthy in time.

Baking Soda Toothpaste

At one point it seemed every company jumped on the baking soda toothpaste bandwagon! Baking soda in paste form goes back to 1917, when a company first produced toothpaste containing this healthful ingredient. Baking soda has value because it neutralizes the acid produced by bacteria. Because baking soda is sold in powder form, people think it is an abrasive product; but in fact, it is low in abrasive properties. Just as it can be placed in the refrigerator to absorb bacteria, so it can be placed in your mouth to achieve the same effect. Additionally, as it is an antacid, it can neutralize the acids in your mouth that can irritate gum tissue and cause mouth malodor (bad breath) and decay.

Tea Tree Oil Toothpaste

Toothpaste with tea tree oil can be antiseptic, as this oil has antibacterial, antiviral, and antifungal properties. Do not use this product every day, as I find that toothpaste with these components can irritate the gum tissue if used daily.

Aloe Vera Gel

Aloe vera can be used in gel toothpaste. It speeds the healing of damaged tissue and can be spread on the toothbrush to massage the gums. It has a slight numbing effect, so it can be soothing if your teeth are supersensitive. You can also massage your gums with the gel. The gum tissue needs to be nurtured and cleansed in a different way than the structure of teeth. The tooth structure is made of minerals, and the gum tissue is made up of cells, much like the skin on your face. Aloe vera gel is used primarily for the skin but can be used for the gums as an emollient (softener) and can help moisturize the gum tissue. This is a good product for mouth breathers.

Myrrh Toothpaste

Myrrh is a powerful antiseptic and often is used in natural toothpaste. I have found, however, that if you use this daily, the gums become irritated. Myrrh may be too be caustic, even though it is considered holistic in nature. So only use myrrh if an area of your mouth is inflamed. Do not use this product daily. Weleda brand makes a pink toothpaste with myrrh in it, and many people like the taste and color of the toothpaste. Frequent use can become a problem for people sensitive to myrrh. If your gums get irritated by using it on a daily basis, alternate your toothpaste. You can use different herbal toothpastes much the same way you would change your skin care products and shampoos from day to day.

Calendula Toothpaste

Calendula toothpaste is a natural toothpaste that can act as a homeopathic antiseptic. Calendula, also known as marigold, is an annual herb that helps reduce gum disease naturally. It works well with echinacea toothpaste.

Propolis Toothpaste

Propolis is a sticky substance gathered by bees from the leaves and bark of trees. Bees use this substance to form the walls of their hives. Propolis has astonishing antibiotic properties and is highly effective against infections in the mouth. It is an excellent substance in reversing gum disease. It has anti-inflammatory agents, and contains traces of minerals vital to healthy bone for the support of your teeth. It not only acts as a powerful local antiseptic that soothes, but it has a mild local anesthetic effect that accelerates healing. Toothpaste containing propolis is useful in fighting off infections caused by periodontal disease.

Chew Stick Toothpaste (Peelu)

Recently, chew sticks used in developing countries to clean the teeth have been treated pharmaceutically to produce a pleasant, natural toothpaste. In various parts of the world such as the West Indies and Africa, the chew stick is picked from trees. Natives chew at the end of the stick until a fiber brush is formed, which produces a bitter, cleansing foam. The foam can be swallowed or spat out. The minerals from the stick are natural and healthy for the teeth, gums, and body. I suggest that you spit out the foam. Native peoples who still use chew sticks today are noted for white, sparkling teeth and healthy gums. They rarely show dental decay.

Seeds, Berries, and Leaves

Seeds

Sesame and sunflower seeds have minerals needed for strong teeth and healthy gums. Chew them slowly, and you will find that they help strengthen the gum tissue.

Berries

Bilberries are a fruit that can help in dental hygiene. The American blueberry is the same as the European bilberry, a perennial shrub that grows in Europe. The major difference between the two is that the American blueberry is white or cream-colored inside, while the European bilberry is purple. Bilberries and bilberry extract can be found in health food stores. Berries have an astringent and antiseptic effect on the mouth, and help in reducing infections due to gum disease. They help in circulation and healing tissue. Take a mouthful of bilberries and chew them very, very slowly. Then expel them if you want. Bilberries and many other berries are rich sources of minerals, vitamin C, and beta-carotine, as well as flavonoids and other compounds that have a marked antiseptic action. If you eat them slowly, the nutrients will be absorbed by the tissue. Other berries good for gum tissue are strawberries, black currants, and cherries. Blackberries are known to heal teeth and gums. Many people in the old days drank blackberry tea for healthier gums and teeth. Blackberry is known for its tonic, antiseptic, and regenerative action on the mucous membranes of the mouth.

Leaves

House leek leaves are also astringent and healing. Try chewing a leaf and keeping it in your mouth for a few minutes. You can get these leaves in the health food store. Olive leaves are a Mediterranean remedy used for bleeding and infected gums. Simmer a small pinch of olive leaves in water for about twenty minutes. Cool, strain, and then use as a mouth rinse. This olive juice, mixed half and half with distilled water, makes an excellent mouthwash.

Toothbrushes

Natural toothbrushes can be used in place of nylon tooth-brushes. In other parts of the world, many people use healing plants and twigs (like the chew stick) that provide a natural-bristle, disposable brush that promotes healing.

However, there is no one ideal toothbrush, since what's important is the technique. The natural process of massage is the important factor here. Massage stimulates gum tissue and brings healing cells to the surface. Gum tissue is treated in much the same way as the skin on your face. The natural process of healing comes from stimulating the blood cells by massage.

Tinctures

You can buy tinctures in most health food stores. You may also find tinctures in health food catalogues. If you have any problems locating them, just write to me (see address at the back of the book) and I can order them for you. Tinctures are made from herbs and can be used at home. Add the tincture to an oral irrigator and then irrigate the tincture mixed with water onto and under the gums. When I treat patients' gum tissues by deep root planing and scaling, I dip the instrument into the tinctures and also use a sponge applicator to place the tincture into the affected gum pocket. After the tincture is placed in the pocket, I massage the gum tissue to help it absorb the tincture.

Calendula Tincture

Calendula is an herb that has a wonderful effect on chronic gum disease. If your gums are continuously bleeding, you can try using calendula in a tincture form. Place two or three drops of it under your tongue. There are two other ways to apply the tincture directly to the gum tissue. Put some herbal toothpaste on a toothbrush, then put two drops of the tincture directly on the paste. Then brush, massaging the toothpaste and the tincture into the gum tissue. You can also place the tincture into the gum pocket through an irrigation system (see page 94). Following the placement of the tincture, take your toothbrush and massage the tincture into the tissue. The gum will then heal and the tissue will revitalize.

Chamomile Tincture

Chamomile is another tincture that can be used to recondition the tissue. The most familiar and common varieties of chamomile are matricaria and German. This annual plant grows in uncultivated fields among wheat and corn, especially in the sandy regions of Europe. Use the chamomile tincture the same as you would a calendula tincture or any other tincture. It is a good anti-inflammatory.

Echinacea Tincture

Echinacea is often called coneflower, and is found in the Great Plains region of North America. Echinacea acts as an external wound healer and an anti-inflammatory. Echinacea is beneficial to use for gum disease and should be placed under the gum either with a sponge applicator, or with your toothbrush topped with toothpaste that has the tincture added to it.

Goldenseal Tincture

Goldenseal stimulates the immune system and is considered to be an antimicrobial remedy. It is effective in fighting bacteria strains such as staphylococcus and streptococcus, among others. Use in the same way as echinacea.

Cayenne Tincture

Cayenne pepper, or red pepper, acts as a stimulant and is good for receding (shrinking) gums. It also brings blood flow into the area of an infection. Use on occasion, in the same way as echinacea.

Propolis Tincture

Propolis is a natural antibacterial tincture and should be used for gum problems. However, it has a thick composition, which can make the applicator sticky. If placed directly on the toothpaste, it may make the brush thick and sticky, so use a separate brush to apply this tincture.

Oral Irrigators

Oral irrigators, such as the Water Pik, can aid in directing natural healing products under the gum and into the pocket of the gum. Using pure distilled water in the oral irrigator with a natural antibacterial such as the extracts mentioned above will help fight gum disease and reverse the process naturally. But it is important to remember to use these tools daily. Using an oral irrigator is like washing your skin. A tincture will not clog your oral irrigator, but if it seems sluggish, flush it out with warm water and vinegar.

Follow these instructions carefully for oral irrigation:

1. Use low to medium pressure. When the gums feel strong, you can raise the pressure a small amount. Most irrigation systems have numbers—do not exceed number five on the system.
2. Use warm water. Water that is too hot or too cold in the oral irrigator can cause gum irritation.
3. Fill the base with distilled water and then add two or three capfuls of peroxide or echinacea mouthwash; or, if you have a battery-operated oral irrigator, you can use baking soda or salt. The amount of mouthwash you should add is a few capfuls; the same goes for salt or baking soda.
4. Work around the gum line at a right angle. Hold the pick at a right angle. Wherever the gums seem to be weak and irritated, go over that area lightly; and return again at the end to go over the weakened area. Never abuse the tissue—listen to your body and work gently. Too many people think they are removing caverns of food—it is more important that you irrigate carefully.
5. Use the entire reservoir, and if needed, fill again.

It is important to irrigate your teeth at night because bacteria manifest quicker at night as the metabolic system relaxes. You also have less saliva at night, making it easier for bacteria to invade the gum tissue.

Orangewood Sticks

Orangewood sticks are great interdental cleansing tools. The orangewood is a natural wood that is softer than a regular toothpick. The orangewood can massage the soft, fragile gum tissue while cleaning between the teeth.

Rubber Points or Tips

Massage of the gums can be done naturally with the rubber pointed tips of your toothbrush, or a separate tipped instrument. The rubber tip can shrink the swollen gum found between the teeth.

Aromatherapy and Its Use in Gum Therapy

The aromas of flower and herb essences have healing effects on the body. This can be related to the mind-body healing system. Have you noticed that some scents make you feel good and that you are repelled by others? Aromatherapy can be used either in private practice or in your home. Aromatherapy uses essential oils to aid in healing. These oils are the natural distilled essences of plants, herbs, and flowers—considered to be the heart and soul of the plant.

For most of us, eucalyptus may have been our first connection to aromatherapy. Do you remember having a cold and having had Vicks VapoRub rubbed onto your chest? The massage may have felt good and opened your sinuses, but more important, you *felt* better. The eucalyptus used in VapoRub is one of the essential oils. Eucalyptus can energize you, and you can awaken the senses readily with this aroma. It is also used for opening the passages to the sinus cavities, reducing any tendency to breathe through the mouth.

Some oils, including lavender, chamomile, and rose, are calming. Lavender relaxes the body. Used in the evening, it can even help you sleep. I personally use lavender oil on the inside of my hands when I work on patients. This expedites the healing process that I am trying to achieve on the gum tissue. I also have a candle lit with the essence of lavender inside it. While we all know that a dental office does not have the reputation for being relaxing, I can't get my patients out of the chair when I use aromatherapy to help heal their gums!

Essential oils act on the adrenals, ovaries, and other organs. Since they can energize, pacify, detoxify, and work on the digestive system, they are an aid to healing gum tissue. Each oil's therapeutic properties also make it effective for treating gum infections, as well as infection in other parts of the body. These oils are also mood regulators and can enhance your immune system by elevating your mood. The different essences can control heart rate, blood pressure, breathing, memory, and stress levels, too. When the essential oils help elevate your mood and reduce anxiety, they reduce the need for antidepressants, which may cause dry mouth and toxicity. All this helps your chances of reversing gum disease naturally.

Essential oils can be applied in a massage, used in a bath, inhaled in steam, and sprayed into the air. In Europe, they are prescribed by doctors for their patients. The cost of essential oils varies tremendously, ranging from $3 a half ounce for some citrus fragrances to $400 or more for rose oil. The prices are so high for rose essence because it takes thousands of rose petals to generate a tiny amount of rose oil, whereas citrus products are plentiful and their oil is easy to extract.

Aromatherapy in the Home for Gum Care

Aromatherapy is ideal for home use. Most health food stores carry a wide variety of essential oils. The following are some ideas on how to use these essential oils at home for gum care.

- *Daily hygiene:* Gentle oils such as *eucalyptus radiata, niaouli,* and *ravensara aromatica* can be used on the skin before or after a shower. Put lavender oil on your wrists when you start your daily hygiene routine, especially in the evening, to enhance healing of the gum tissue.
- *Stress:* A drop of anise oil with a spoonful of honey helps to relieve gastrointestinal cramping. Stress can be a major cause of gum disease, and anise oil will help soothe your intestinal system and increase your body's chances to fight off gum disease.
- *Energy:* Most of us need more energy in the morning and evening. Black spruce and peppermint are effective stimulants that work by strengthening the adrenal cortex. The resulting energy will then enhance your hygiene routine and boost your immune system so that it fights off disease and infection. It will also stimulate the blood flow to bring the gum tissue to a healthier state.
- *Relaxation:* Essential oils, such as lavender or chamomile, can be diffused in the air. Buy a diffuser and place the essential oils on the heated tray to have the essence diffused in the air to create a relaxing atmosphere. Lavender oil added to the bath or sprayed in

your bedroom will relax you during sleep. The deep body relaxation afforded by sleep is imperative to healing any of your body parts, including your gums.

Various Essential Oils

Mandarin Oil

Mandarin oil is especially good to use with young children, as it helps to relax them. If your children are relaxed, you are more apt to be relaxed. Mandarin can also reduce anxiety for adults, thus creating a more positive outlook and helping your gums to heal faster.

Chamomile Oil

This oil will calm an upset mind or tense body. A drop or two rubbed on the solar plexus can reduce the tense and upset parts of your body.

Rosemary Oil

This oil has similar benefits to those of toothpaste because it activates the metabolism in the outer layer of the skin and improves cell regeneration needed for healthy gums.

Geranium Oil

This is an oil with antifungal and antiviral properties. It is gentle to the skin and can be used for topical application.

Holistic therapies, which include holistic products, help access the body's healing potential. Many of these natural herbs are old remedies that have been rediscovered to enhance the natural healing processes of the gums. Herbs have always been integral to the practice of medicine, and modern medicine uses plants in pharmaceutical medicine. It is interesting to note that in modern medicine, pure herbs are rarely used, probably due to the fact that you cannot patent a natural product.

However, the demand for natural, holistic care products has been increasing. Even though it is an old treatment method, it is rarely used in modern medicine, and is even less common in the prevention of gum disease. Many health food stores now have their shelves stocked with natural herbal products, but it has been only in the last five years that these products have become available in commercial drug chains.

6

Therapeutic Healing

The mouth needs nurturing and healing products to induce a natural reversal of gum disease. Unfortunately, many of us take out our anger on our teeth's fragile gum tissue. (If you realize this, then you are already ahead of the game.) Oral therapeutics, however, strive for healing of the gum tissue. Healing of any tissue of the body needs proper guidance with the right products, and most of all, our own loving touch.

"Therapeutics" refers to energy transference and is simply the use of heart energy. We use the energy of our hearts when we love to do something—such as eating a certain food, loving a person, or even caring for an animal or plant. This nurturing and heart energy combine to create a therapeutic effect.

Therapeutic touch is used as an energy healing system in many American medical facilities and hospitals. It operates on the premise that the healing force of the therapist affects the healing force within the patient. Yet healing through the use of therapeutics has rarely been discussed for general mouth care, although the soft tissues of the gum can be an indicator in the healing arts. You can see changes in the body by the condition of the gums. As discussed in chapter 2, the mouth is a mirror of the body. Western energy therapies aim to balance a person's energy through touch. Transferring energy from one's hands to the area that needs healing can reduce pain and aid the dental practitioner in being able to work deeper into the gum pocket without causing the patient too much pain.

Healing therapeutics can even be used by you, when you are massaging your gums with a toothbrush. The healing, loving touch of your hands on the brush offers the energy needed for you to heal your gums naturally. Read on! You will learn how therapeutic energy is used to heal your mouth.

Therapeutic Healing Used for the Natural Reversal of Gum Disease

In dentistry, and especially in dental hygiene, the myriad of products available to cleanse and cure our mouth and any problems seem to focus on bacterial plaque. But is there another aspect we are leaving out, especially when we remember that gum tissue connects to the total body? Margins of crowns and bridges can cause loose and swollen tissue. Stress itself is the most prominent reason for loose, baggy gums.

Energetic Relations of Teeth with Organs of the Body

There is a theory that the teeth relate energetically to the organs. Reflexology is the study of the meridians that connect to the bodily organs in an organic totality; the mouth is included in this. The meridians are energetic pathways between the teeth and the organs. Meridians surround each tooth, connecting them to the total body. For example, the upper right wisdom tooth relates to the anterior pituitary lobe, internal ear, tongue, shoulder, top of the foot, sacroiliac joint, duodenum on the right side, and central nervous system. The upper left first molar relates energetically to the thyroid, parathyroid, tongue, mandibular sinus, spleen, esophagus, and the stomach on the left side. The lower right central tooth relates energetically to the following parts and organs: rectum, bladder, kidney on the right side, genitourinary area, posterior knee, sacrococcygeal joint, ankle joint posterior, nose, and adrenal gland. For more about such connections, see the following chart. The right and left teeth do not necessary respond to the right and left of each organ.

Energetic Relations of Teeth in Relationship with Organs and Tissues of the Total Body

Upper Teeth

Tooth #1 (upper right third molar—wisdom tooth): anterior pituitary lobe, internal ear, tongue, sacroiliac joint, foot plantar side, shoulder, heart right side, duodenum right side, terminal ileum, central nervous system

(continues)

Energetic Relations of Teeth *(continued)*

Tooth #2 (upper right second molar): parathyroid, thyroid, tongue, maxillary sinus, jaw, anterior hip, anterior knee, medial ankle joint, pancreas, esophagus right side, mammary gland right side

Tooth #3 (upper right first molar): parathyroid, thyroid, tongue, maxillary sinus, jaw, anterior hip, anterior knee, medial ankle joint, pancreas, esophagus right side, mammary gland right side

Tooth #4 (upper right second bicuspid): thymus, posterior pituitary, nose, ethmoid cells, front big toe, lung right side, large intestine right side, mammary gland right side

Tooth #5 (upper right first bicuspid): thymus, posterior pituitary, nose, ethmoid cells, front big toe, lung right side, large intestine right side

Tooth #6 (cuspid): intermediate pituitary lobe, hip, lateral ankle joint, liver right side, gall bladder right side

Tooth #7 (lateral incisor): pineal gland, nose, sphenoidal sinus, posterior knee, posterior ankle joint, kidney right side, bladder right side, genitourinary area, rectum

Tooth #8 (central incisor): pineal gland, nose, frontal sinus, sacrococcygeal joint, posterior ankle joint, kidney right side, bladder right side, genitourinary area, rectum

Tooth #9 (left central incisor): pineal gland, nose, sphenoidal sinus, frontal sinus, posterior knee, sacrococcygeal joint, posterior ankle joint, kidney left side, bladder left side, genitourinary area, rectum

Tooth #10 (upper left lateral incisor): pineal gland, nose, sphenoidal sinus, frontal sinus, posterior knee, sacrococcygeal joint, ankle joint posterior, kidney left side, bladder left side, genitourinary area, rectum

Tooth #11 (upper left cuspid): posterior pituitary lobe, eye posterior portion, sphenoidal sinus, hip, lateral ankle joint, liver left side, biliary ducts left side

Tooth #12 (upper left first bicuspid): intermediate posterior pituitary lobe, nose, ethmoid cells, shoulder/elbow, hand radial side, lung left side, large intestine left side

Tooth #13 (upper left second bicuspid): thymus, nose, ethmoid cells, shoulder/elbow, hand radial side, lung left side, large intestine left side

Tooth #14 (upper left first molar): thyroid, tongue, maxillary sinus, jaw, anterior hip, anterior knee, medial ankle joint, spleen, esophagus, stomach left side

Tooth #15 (upper left second molar): parathyroid, tongue, maxillary sinus, jaw, anterior hip, anterior knee, medial ankle joint, spleen, esophagus, stomach left side

Tooth #16 (upper left third molar—wisdom tooth): anterior pituitary lobe, internal ear, tongue, foot plantar side, shoulder/elbow, hand, sacroiliac joint, heart left side, duodenum left side, central nervous system

Lower Teeth

Tooth #17 (lower left third molar—wisdom tooth): peripheral nerves, ileum left side, heart left side, shoulder/elbow left side, hand, toes, sacroiliac joint, middle external ear, tongue

Tooth #18 (lower left second molar): arteries, large intestine left side, lung left side, shoulder/elbow left side, hand, foot, big toe, ethmoid cells, nose

(continues)

Energetic Relations of Teeth *(continued)*

Tooth #19 (lower left first molar): veins, large intestine left side, lung left side, shoulder/elbow left side, hand, big toe, ethmoid cells, nose

Tooth #20 (lower left second bicuspid): mammary glands, lymph vessels, esophagus, stomach left side, spleen, anterior hip, anterior knee, medial ankle joint, maxillary sinus, tongue, gonad

Tooth #21 (lower left first bicuspid): mammary glands, lymph vessels, esophagus, stomach left side, spleen, anterior hip, anterior knee, medial ankle joint, maxillary sinus, tongue, gonad

Tooth #22 (lower left cuspid): biliary ducts left side, liver left side, hip, sphenoidal sinus, eye anterior portion, gonad

Tooth #23 (lower left lateral incisor): rectum, anal canal, bladder left side, genitourinary area, kidney left side, posterior knee, ankle joint, frontal sinus, nose, adrenal glands

Tooth #24 (lower left central incisor): rectum, anal canal, bladder left side, genitourinary area, kidney left side, posterior knee, ankle joint, frontal sinus, nose, adrenal glands

Tooth #25 (lower right central incisor): rectum, anal canal, genitourinary area, kidney right side, posterior knee, ankle joint posterior, frontal sinus, sphenoidal sinus, nose, adrenal glands

Tooth #26 (lower right central incisor): rectum, anal canal, genitourinary area, kidney right side, posterior knee, ankle joint posterior, frontal sinus, sphenoidal sinus, nose, adrenal glands

Tooth #27 (lower right central incisor): gall bladder, biliary ducts right side, liver right side, posterior knee, lateral ankle joint, frontal sinus, sphenoidal sinus, eye anterior position, gonad

Tooth #28 (lower right first bicuspid): esophagus/stomach right side, pylorus pyloric antrum, pancreas, anterior hip, anterior knee, medial ankle joint, jaw, maxillary sinus, tongue, gonad

Tooth #29 (lower right second bicuspid): lymph vessels, esophagus/stomach right side, pylorus pyloric antrum, pancreas, anterior hip, anterior knee, medial ankle joint, jaw, maxillary sinus, tongue

Tooth #30 (lower right first molar): veins, large intestine right side, lung right side, shoulder/elbow right side, hand radial side, foot, big toe, ethmoid cells, nose

Tooth #31 (lower right second molar): arteries, large intestine right side, shoulder/elbow right side, hand radial side, foot, big toe, ethmoid cells, nose

Tooth #32 (lower right third molar): peripheral nerves, terminal deum, heart right side, shoulder/elbow right side, hand, ulnar side, foot plantar side, toes, sacroiliac joint, middle ear, tongue

Good clinical skills are needed for your gums to heal correctly. If you go for a routine cleaning, make sure that your practitioner chooses a soft, therapeutic approach to clean the tartar away and restore the health of your gum tissue. Using high-tech instruments to remove diseased tissue may be an easier approach for a dental practitioner, but it should not replace the therapeutic approach or good-quality hand scaling. And while it is important to remove the diseased tissue, it is *more* important to obtain reattachment after the diseased tissue is removed. Using therapeutics in dental hygiene can help enhance this healing process.

But you do not have to depend on someone else for a healing therapeutic touch. Tissue control starts with good manual dexterity—an ability also needed when you massage your gums with your brush. As you know, therapeutic healing is the transference of healing energy from your hands to the area that needs healing. How do you go about doing this?

First, if you love what you are doing, then you will do it well, and the extra heart-filled or healing energy will help you to reverse your gum condition naturally. How many people just brush their teeth because they know they have to? How many really "get into" the brushing of their teeth? A dentist I know says he loves to brush his teeth and massage his gums. It takes him approximately four minutes in the morning and four minutes in the evening. Do you feel this way about brushing your teeth and massaging your gums? If you don't, it's time to change how you feel. Are you using healing therapeutic arts to reverse your gum disease naturally? Now that you have become aware that using extra heart (therapeutic) energy will help heal your gum tissue, you will be able to start to work more efficiently with your brush.

So nurture your fragile gum tissue. Using therapeutic touch on your mouth will also help you to energize your entire body. Sloppy, routine brushing will not do the job. Whatever time you spend, do it with heart-filled energy and the results will be very rewarding. It is hard to practice such self-massage on your entire body, but using it to massage your gums is quite easy. When massaging your gums, become aware of the healing energy we all produce. This energy can be used by each and every individual. Tap into the greatest source of energy: your own.

Understanding the importance of therapeutics will then help you develop a positive approach to oral hygiene habits. Feel the results! Your mouth will be energized. This is the feeling you want when you wake in the morning. You'll no longer notice a dry, foul odor in your mouth. Here are some tools that use the power of touch and contact to bring healing energy to the gums.

Using Therapeutic Healing with Oral Care Products

Toothbrush Massage

Massage is mostly thought of as a total body workout. The gum tissue needs similar treatment. Think of the fragile tissue as loose flabby muscles. Tightening this loose gum tissue can be done with massage. Massage brings circulation and new blood cells to the area of inflammation. In gum disease, you may find swollen, infected tissue that needs repair and reattachment. The best method of creating healing for the gum tissue is a gentle massage with a soft toothbrush. Cooking has taken us to processed food and soft gourmet eating—but our gums need a workout that soft foods will not provide.

So transfer your energy from your *chi* center into your hands. *Chi* is an energy that we all have. *Chi* is the central concept of Chinese medicine—it means air, vapor, breath, ether, energy; also temperament, strength, atmosphere as

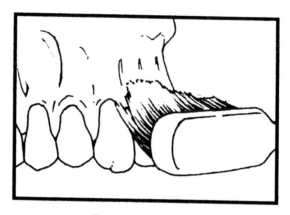

Toothbrush massage.

taken from the center of the being (person). It is also therapeutic energy. *Chi* energy is almost always used when heart
energy is activated. If you merely brush your teeth without
your heart energy, your results will be lessened. Loving what
you do has great results. Calculated cooking, lovemaking, or
oral hygiene will not have the same results as when you love
to cook, put your heart into lovemaking, and as important,
love taking care of your mouth.

How do you get motivated to love your teeth and brush
with heart energy? *Feel!* Learn how it feels when you tap
into heart energy. Stimulate the gum tissue. Massage the
gums instead of merely thinking about the angle of the
brush. In my profession as a dental hygienist, we are told to
tell you to brush at a certain angle. Periodically we direct
patients to brush at a different angle. Rhythm also has a therapeutic effect on the mouth, so try to brush with rhythm.

The *chi,* or life-sustaining force, is in everyone. If you
work technically and are not using your inner *chi* energy,

then you will get mechanical results. The healing power of *chi* is in all of us—use it! The healing therapeutic touch will be transferred from your hands through the brush to the gum tissue to heal and tighten against the bone. Feel the energy flow throughout your mouth. If you notice a little blood on the brush, let it be a diagnostic indicator that this area needs more healing and massage. And be gentle with yourself, love your mouth, and most important, love yourself. If you are massaging your gums in the evening, make sure to softly massage the tissue resting against the bony structures of your teeth. Think about how you are reattaching loosened tissue as you have worked your teeth and gums all day by eating, drinking, and talking.

Oral Irrigator

Use an oral irrigator to massage the gum pocket. The oral irrigator will not only irrigate the particles of food out

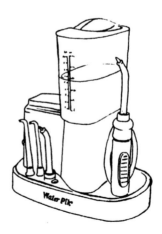

Oral irrigator.

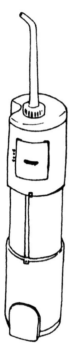

Electric oral irrigator, portable.

from under your gums, but will work your gums with massage therapy. Think of a shower massage working your back muscles—the same can be done for your gums. Use the oral irrigator on a low to medium pressure. Too high a pressure can rip the gum tissue and cause infection and damage.

Also, an oral irrigator, manual or electric, has a force of water released from the hose. This water can direct antibacterial agents or herbs under the gum. The release of antibacterial agents and herbs through the oral irrigator will thus create healing. As the healing system also depends on good blood circulation, an oral irrigator (as well as a toothbrush) can stimulate the proper circulation through massage.

Rubber Tip Stimulator

Another way to massage the gums is with a rubber tip. Using a rubber tip with rhythm can heal the gum tissue. You can tighten the gums with a circular motion of the rubber tip. Point the rubber tip toward the incisor (top) edge of your teeth. Then work the rubber tip around the gums using your natural rhythm.

A rubber tip will also aid in bringing circulation to the gum tissue. Using a rubber tip stimulator will bring the healing blood cells to the surface and also enable you to tighten the loose gum tissue that is found in between your teeth.

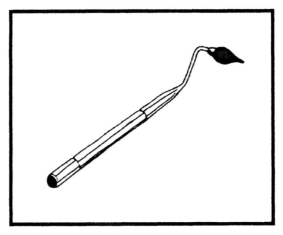

Rubber tip stimulator.

Floss

Floss, when used correctly, can also energize the gum tissue. It can massage away the plaque and food particles. But be sure not to snap the floss! Work the floss around each tooth with rhythm. "Rhythm" is the key word. By using rhythm you release your own therapeutic healing energy. This transference of energy can then be directed onto the gum tissue. Make a "C" shape with the floss and wrap it around each tooth. Slide the floss out and then take a new spot on the floss. Do not use the same piece of floss from one tooth to another, and slide the floss out. Do not pull up or down with the floss, as you may dislodge a filling or a crown, which can be very costly to replace.

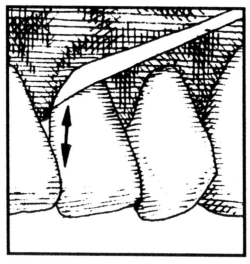

Flossing correctly.

Mouthwash

Bacteria that festers in the mouth are a negative energy form. This negative source of energy can cause mouth malodor (bad breath). The mouthwash you select can rid the mouth of the festering bacteria. Make sure there is an herb in the mouthwash to energize and create circulation for the gums and the surrounding mucous membranes. Herbs play an important role in feeding energy to the tissues. Using herbal mouthwash rinses away the bacteria while feeding and nourishing the cells.

Toothpicks (Orangewood, Plastic)

Toothpicks come in different forms. In a soft orangewood stick, the toothpick can create massage in between the teeth. The papilla (V-shaped gum) can be cleansed with the orangewood stick. You can also use a plastic pick to rid your teeth of plaque before it forms tartar. These picks are

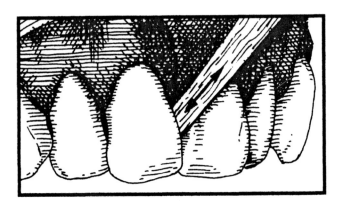

Orangewood stick.

therapeutic and help stimulate the gum tissue. So massage your gums with a wooden stick. Using an orangewood stick, work the stick under the gum, massaging in between your teeth and the gum line.

Toothpaste

Herbal and antibacterial toothpaste can be listed among the products that are dental therapeutics. Toothpaste with the proper ingredients, such as mint and rosemary, can cause the gums to be stimulated and massaged. Echinacea toothpaste will help to therapeutically heal gum tissue. Antibacterial agents such as baking soda will help balance the pH of the mouth.

What about Electric Toothbrushes?

Circulation of the gum tissue provides a good supply of blood to the tissue. Toughening and increasing the circulation of the gum tissue will reverse gum disease in a natural way. It can help to tighten the tissue and bring the proper source of blood to the inflamed site.

If you choose to massage with a new, high-tech toothbrush, it can help shrink the swollen tissue. Many of these new products have a massage action to the brush. But do not let the brush control you. *You* must control the brush and use your *own* energy to massage with an electric toothbrush. So shimmy an electric toothbrush from side to side. Direct the brush onto the gum tissue. If you hold the brush and let the energy of the brush work without your own energy, it will be less effective.

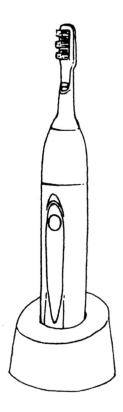

Electric toothbrush.

Healing energy exists for everyone, and you must tap into it. Think of something that flourished because you took loving care of it. It can be a flowering plant or a pet. You probably used heart energy (healing energy) to enhance the growth of this living being. You can use the same heart energy to heal yourself. It can work wonders on gum tissue.

Visualization can also be helpful. If you visualize a white light and see that white light as healing energy, you can transmit that light to the spot you wish to heal. Look at your gum tissue and then visualize a white light of healing energy being sent from your hands to the brush and then directed onto the gum tissue. See yourself heal, and your gum tissue will reverse from disease to health. Feed your gum tissue with healing energy.

7

Diet and Supplements

While the main causes of periodontal disease are stress and
poor oral hygiene, another problem leading to gum disease
may be poor diet. It is the missing link to prevention and
treatment of gum disease, and it is almost always ignored. In
this chapter, I will discuss the need to eat a proper balanced
diet. I will list some foods that will enable you to build
stronger bones and healthier gum tissue.

Why Diet Plays an Important Role

Diet is important in controlling periodontal disease because
bacteria in the mouth use sugars for energy and reproduc-
tion. When your oral hygiene is poor and your diet is high
in sugar, more bacteria are produced. The higher bacterial
level will then inflame the gums and may increase plaque

formation, resulting in gum disease. If we consume a high-sugar diet, the body will produce more bacteria in the mouth. Stress, combined with such a sugar diet, adds acid to our saliva and will show its results in gum disease. (It also may lead to hypoglycemia.) Studies have shown that it is more harmful to eat sugar-containing foods between meals than it is to eat them with meals.

We need vitamins and minerals in our diet. Vitamins help regulate our metabolism. A diet high in fiber and fruits and vegetables will help to reverse gum problems naturally. Most important, we need the fats and proteins that provide the energy that helps build the cells of our body. To reverse gum disease naturally, we must alter our diet and discipline ourselves to maintain healthier eating patterns. Please see a nutritionist to get counseling for a diet that is programmed for you specifically.

In isolated areas where groups of aboriginal people live, it has been proven that their teeth and gums are in a healthy state. These groups do not follow what we consider proper oral hygiene, yet they have healthy mouths. Why? They eat live foods and basically lead simple, stress-free lives. If these people came to live here, their teeth and gums would start to show disease states that would be due to the processed foods that we eat.

People who are obese and eat sugary foods have a higher susceptibility to gum disease than those who eat a balanced diet. Soft and sticky food (like nutrition bars), which tend to remain in the grooves of the teeth, are also a culprit and can lead to tooth and gum problems. It is not the vitamin content but the natural sugars such as honey in these nutritional bars that get stuck in the grooves of your teeth.

Is it true that what we are is what we eat? Yes! I hope that after reading this chapter you will begin to eat a balanced diet, and to try to consume the recommended daily allowances of nutrients as suggested by the U.S. Department of Agriculture.

Caution: Certain medications and conditions alter vitamin and mineral balance. See a nutritionist or internist for individual guidance.

Vitamins

Vitamin A

The bone surrounding the teeth needs attention given to it that is equal to that given to other bones in the body. Vitamin A is needed for the formation of this bone.

Vitamin A deficiency in the mouth can show up as thin enamel, chalky patches on your teeth, decreased tooth growth, retarded eruption, malpositioned teeth, soft teeth, dry mouth, and defective dentin formation, because it can decrease the activity of new cells. On the other hand, excessive consumption of vitamin A can result in a toxic condition characterized by itching skin, gum disease (gingivitis), and irritability. Other physical symptoms may manifest, such as poor night vision, lack of appetite and vigor, bladder stones, and hyperthyroidism. Note: If you have any of the symptoms listed, consult your medical doctor or see a nutritionist.

Too much or too little can affect your teeth and gums. Eating foods such as the following, in moderation, will help you to heal your mouth and reverse your gum condition. The soft foods containing vitamin A that are easier on the teeth are foods like apricot and cantaloupes. Harder foods include carrots, broccoli, and celery. Additional foods containing vitamin A are alfalfa, amaranth fruit, asparagus, basil, beans, beet greens, butter, cabbage, carrot tops, chicory, chilis, chives, egg yolk, elderberry, endive, escarole, and milk.

Recommended daily intake: 5,000 IU for men, 4,000 IU for women, 5,000 IU for pregnant women, and 700 IU for children.

Vitamin B

If you have a vitamin B deficiency, your tongue may show some early symptoms of enlarged taste buds (bumps on the top of your tongue) at the front and the side, with the taste buds in the back of your tongue becoming enlarged later on. You also may also notice deep fissures and grooves down the center of the tongue. Various foods fit in different vitamin B groups. Foods that are high in vitamin B include mushrooms, algae, yeast, sunflower seeds, and sesame seeds.

Vitamin B₁ (Thiamin)

Thiamin was the first B vitamin discovered; this is why it is designated as vitamin B_1. Symptoms of a severe deficiency of vitamin B_1 include a burning sensation on the tongue, loss of taste, unusual sensitivity of the inner lining (the cheeks and soft tissue) of the mouth, and cracks and sores in the corner of the mouth. Cracks in the corner of the mouth, called "angular cheilosis," are common. Foods rich in vitamin B_1 that can help you avoid such symptoms are wheat, bran, oatmeal, legumes such as peanuts, and peas. Meat, fish, fruit, and milk also contain thiamin.

Recommended daily intake: 1.1 to 1.4 mg for adults, and 1.2 mg for children.

Vitamin B_2 (Riboflavin)

This vitamin is involved in the production of energy through the conversion of nutrients in food. Commonly, symptoms of riboflavin deficiency are lips that may crack and become painful and ulcerated. They appear redder or whiter than usual. The corners of the mouth may also crack. Contact with food or drink may cause pain or a burning sensation on the tongue. Antidepressants decrease the positive effect of this vitamin, so be especially watchful if you are being treated for depression. Food rich in vitamin B_2 are brewer's yeast, calves' liver, almonds, wheat germ, wild rice, soy flour, wheat bran, soybeans (raw), sunflower seeds, prunes, beans, and peas.

Recommended daily intake: 1.2 to 1.7 mg for adults, and 1.4 mg for children.

Vitamin B_3 (Niacin)

Niacin is involved in the metabolism of carbohydrates and fats. It acts as a coenzyme (catalyst) in the process that requires energy for normal cell function. Vitamin B_3 deficiency results in pellagra, a disease characterized by a swollen tongue, inflammation of the mouth, diarrhea, and small, red eruptions on the backs of the hands. Good sources of niacin are meats, turkey and other poultry, fish, and peanuts. Fish that are rich in niacin are tuna, salmon, and swordfish. If you have any of the above symptoms and they seem to be lingering, seek the advice of a physician.

Recommended daily intake: 13 to 19 mg for adults, and 16 mg for children.

Vitamin B₅ (Pantothenic Acid)

This vitamin is converted in the body to a catalyst called coenzyme A. The breakdown of fatty acids, metabolism of carbohydrates, conversion of glycogen to glucose, and steroid hormones require coenzyme A. Deficiencies of vitamin B_5 are extremely rare. If this occurs, a person is severely fatigued, and has headaches, nausea, abdominal pain, and cramping of leg muscles. Tobacco use decreases the absorption of this vitamin. Foods rich in this vitamin are brewer's yeast, calves' liver, peanuts, soybean flour, pecans, oatmeal (raw), hazelnuts, brown rice, peppers, wild rice, and kale.

Recommended daily intake: 10 mg for adults, and 5 mg for children.

Vitamin B₆ (Pyridoxine)

Vitamin B_6 is critical in maintaining hormonal balance and proper immune function. In the mouth a sign of its deficiency may be cracking of the lips and tongue.

Vitamin B_6 plays a vital role in the production of new cells, and contributes to a properly functioning immune system. This affects the mouth because it plays an important role in the health of the mucous membranes and skin. These tissues have a great need for the proper amount of vitamin B_6. Low levels of vitamin B_6 (as well as folic acid and vitamin B_{12}) may contribute to osteoporosis. This vitamin thus has an important effect on tissue control and bone loss.

Foods rich in this vitamin are brewer's yeast, sunflower seeds, wheat germ, soybeans, walnuts, soybean flour, lentils, brown rice, hazelnuts, bananas, avocados, whole wheat flour, spinach, potatoes, prunes, raisins, Brussels sprouts, barley, sweet potatoes, and cauliflower.

Recommended daily intake: 1.8 to 2.2 mg for adults, and 1.6 mg for children.

Vitamin B_{12} (Cyanobalmine)

Vitamin B_{12} is found in bacteria that are eaten by animal species, which many of us then end up eating. It is not found in plants, and so getting the proper amount can be a problem for vegetarians. Signs of deficiencies in the mouth are soreness and burning of the tongue and painful, bright red sores that occur on the inner lining of the cheeks and under the surface of the tongue.

Recommended daily intake: 3 micrograms for adults and children.

Vitamin C

Vitamin C is needed for collagen and is needed for building bone cells. Since vitamin C is responsible for the formation of collagen, a constituent of all connective tissue, it is one of the most important vitamins for healthy gums and for proper healing to take place after mouth surgery. Vitamin C deficiency can cause the mouth to be extremely dry, which can lead to tooth decay and gum disease. Because the mouth is a mirror of the body, it may show early signs of vitamin C deficiency, such as bleeding gums. Other symptoms may include too easy bruising.

Foods rich in vitamin C are oranges, grapefruit, honeydew, strawberries, potatoes, and green vegetables.

Recommended daily intake: 60 mg for adults, and 45 to 50 mg for children.

Vitamin D

In a healthy person vitamin D can be synthesized through the skin from cholesterol, which makes this vitamin act more like a hormone, as it aids in the assimilation of calcium. Vitamin D is produced by the interaction of the sun's ultraviolet rays with oils of the skin. The mouth's first symptoms of this deficiency might be excessive tooth decay, and the patient may complain of general weakness. The ultimate vitamin D source is the sun. You can use the skin as an absorptive organ by using unsaturated vegetable oil on the skin (olive or almond oil) and then sunbathing. With the ozone layer thinned, I would suggest that you do not sit in the sun for more then a few minutes. Use caution! Overexposure to the sun can lead to sunburn and possibly even skin cancer. Food products with vitamin D include milk and fish-liver oils.

Recommended daily intake: 400 IU for adults and children.

Vitamin E

Vitamin E is an antioxidant for vitamins A, B, and C, and prevents calcium deposits in blood vessel walls. It also reduces the body's need for oxygen. Vitamin E is found in algae, spirulina, soy, and wheat germ.

Recommended daily intake: 15 to 20 IU for adults, and 9 to 15 IU for children.

Vitamin K

Vitamin K is needed for blood clotting. If your gums bleed and the blood does not coagulate, you may have a vitamin K deficiency. Use of aspirin, mineral oil, antibiotics and sulfa drugs, and exposure to X rays or air pollutants can lead to vitamin K deficiency. Fiber is important in a person's diet, because it is needed for good intestinal motility and it has minerals bound to it (such as calcium pectate).

Food sources rich in vitamin K are chestnuts, spinach, cabbage, cauliflower, seaweed, tomato, broccoli, Brussels sprouts, turnip greens, and lettuce.

Recommended daily intake: 45 to 65 micrograms for adults, and 5 to 30 micrograms for children.

Minerals

Minerals play an important role in dental care because they make teeth harder than bones, which enables you to have stronger teeth for chewing. Most minerals are essential in small amounts but are toxic if too much is ingested. Calcium is the most abundant mineral in the body and makes up to 2 percent of total body weight. Its major function is in building bones, which support the roots of your teeth, and the building of tooth structure. The importance of minerals is to strengthen the teeth and bone support so that your natural teeth will last a lifetime.

Calcium

About one-third of our bones and teeth is made up of calcium. Bone is what is responsible for holding your teeth in place. Calcium also is vitally important for muscle relaxation, acid neutralizing, and blood clotting. A deficiency of calcium might appear as muscle cramps and spasms, and a patient may appear nervous. Foods rich in calcium are acorn, alfalfa, algae, almonds, amaranth, apples, basil, beets, broccoli, cabbage, carob, carrot, dandelion, wheat germ, kelp, macadamia nuts, escarole, custard, olives, orange peel, sesame seeds, sunflower seeds, seaweed, soy, and turnips.

Recommended daily intake: 800 to 1,200 mg for adults and children. It should be increased to 1,600 mg for pregnant and lactating women. If the daily intake of calcium falls below 500 mg, calcium is absorbed from the bones, which makes them more fragile.

Chlorine (Chloride)

Chlorine helps clean out nitrogen and the end products of metabolism. It is responsible for maintaining fluid levels in the body. It also is important for proper digestion. A deficiency of chlorine would show as a loss of hair and teeth. Chronic deficiency also can cause growth failure in children, muscle cramps or weak muscles, mental apathy, loss of appetite, and bad digestion. Foods rich in chlorine are mushrooms, parsley, sweet potato, rhubarb, and *especially* tomato.

Recommended daily intake: No recommended level has been established, but a safe and adequate daily level is estimated at 1,700 to 5,100 mg for adults.

Copper

Copper is needed as an enzyme catalyst. Copper works with iron in the formation of hemoglobin. It also is a product of collagen (connective tissue) and of many enzymes. If there were a deficiency, there would be poor iron assimilation, leading to anemia and scurvylike bone damage. With this deficiency you can have bone loss and resulting gum disease. Foods rich in copper are grains, vegetables, nuts, fish, molasses, raw milk, and fruits.

Recommended daily intake: 1.5 to 3 mg for adults, and 2 to 3 mg for children.

Iron

Iron carries oxygen from the lungs to all the cells. Iron deficiency is most prevalent among women. The tongue may become smooth, giving it a bald appearance. This is due to alterations of the taste buds and the destruction of the papillae surrounding them. A deficiency might appear as fatigue, shortness of breath, or loss of appetite. Iron deficiency can be a contributing factor to gum disease. Seaweed is the richest source of iron, followed by liver, pumpkin and sesame seeds, wheat germ, dried pears and other fruits, nuts, and various kinds of seafood.

Recommended daily intake: 10 to 12 mg for adults, 5 to 10 mg for children, and 10 mg for menopausal women.

Magnesium

Magnesium acts as an important catalyst for many enzymes, and assists in calcium assimilation. It is one of the three most important elements in teeth and bone. The mouth will show deficiencies as slow alveolar bone formation and slow tooth eruption. There may even be gum swelling and weak periodontal fibers. Magnesium deficiency may be indicated by calcium deposits in soft tissue, kidney stones, cramps, hair loss, and irritability.

Foods rich in magnesium are beans (string and kidney), green peas, dried peas, celery, chives, corn, lettuce, orange juice, parsnips, potatoes, radish, rice, scallions, squash, tea (black and green), turnips, malt, peanuts, and tofu.

Recommended daily intake: 350 mg for adults, and 150 mg for children.

Phosphorus

Phosphorus makes up about one-third of bones and teeth. Like calcium, phosphorus is an important element in bone, enamel, and cementum (the layer beneath enamel). If you have a deficiency, you might suffer fatigue and irregular breathing, and have malformed bones. Causes of deficiency might be excessive uses of antacids containing aluminum hydroxide, which inhibits phosphate absorption in the intestine.

Foods rich in phosphorus are malt extract, peanuts, and pecans, as well as pumpkin seeds, brewer's yeast, cheddar cheese, hickory, kelp, Brazil nuts, and wheat germ.

Recommended daily intake: approximately 800 to 1,200 mg for adults, and 150 mg for children.

Selenium

Selenium protects against cadmium and mercury toxicity (including against the mercury in your dental fillings) and overactivity of vitamin E. A deficiency of selenium might show up as aging pigment on your skin. Toxic levels of selenium may cause hair and nail loss, as well as high rates of cavities if selenium was taken during tooth development. Foods rich in selenium are chard, cucumber, fish, pear, sweet potatoes, kidney, liver, and seafood.

Recommended daily intake: Selenium requirements have not been established; adequate amounts are estimated to be 50 to 100 micrograms for adults, and 40 micrograms for children.

Silicon

Silicon is needed for connective tissue, for DNA synthesis, and in maintaining artery walls. It is found in bone-building cells and collagen. It can decrease calcium and increase magnesium in the blood. A silicon deficiency might mean that your bones break more easily. With this deficiency you can have a weaker support of the bone that surrounds the teeth, which is a cause of gum disease. Foods high in silicon are pumpkin, rhubarb, strawberries, and sunflower seeds.

Recommended daily intake: No recommended level has been established.

Sulfur

Sulfur is an important component of the protein chains. It helps the texture and health of the skin and hair, and helps the body to resist bacterial infections, heal wounds, and assimilate other minerals. Foods rich in sulfur are mulberry, parsley, pear, spinach, tomato, turnip, watermelon, Brussels sprouts, dried beans, cabbage, eggs, fish, garlic, and onions.

Recommended daily intake: No recommended allowance has been established.

Zinc

In the human body, zinc is found in all tissues and fluids, but is highly concentrated in teeth, bones, hair, skin, liver, muscle, and testes. Zinc is needed as a catalyst for various enzymes and is part of the hormone insulin. Insulin is secreted in response to high blood sugar as a result of someone ingesting a lot of sugar. This may keep the teeth from receiving this mineral. Zinc influences immune reactions, taste perception, wound healing, and the production of sperm.

A deficiency may result in poor taste and smell, slow wound healing, skeletal defects, white spots on fingernails, thickening and hardening of hair, skin, and arteries, fatigue, and a proneness to infection. This deficiency can be a source of slow healing of the gums, and a cause of gum disease. Foods rich in zinc are goat's milk, monarda, pecans, sweet potato, pumpkin seed, brewer's yeast, green pepper, red meats, shellfish, turkey, and wheat germ.

Recommended daily intake: 15 mg for adults, and 3 to 10 mg for children.

Essential Gum Nutrients

The following are some essential nutrients that can help strengthen your gums. Caution: See an internist or nutritionist because certain medications and illness can affect the dietary intake of vitamins and minerals.

Coenzyme Q_{10}

This vitaminlike substance plays an important role in the energy of each cell. It is claimed to be an antioxidant. Its action in the human body resembles that of vitamin E. Vitamin E helps to preserve CoQ_{10} and is helpful if it is incorporated into the product. Coenzyme Q_{10} is known to combat periodontal disease and can also help with conditions such as allergies, heart disease, diabetes, and asthma. However, I tested some of my patients and did not find that it helped in the improvement or reversal of gum disease. Coenzyme Q_{10} is best absorbed when taking oily foods.

Mackerel, salmon, and sardines contain the largest amounts of CoQ_{10}.

Recommended daily intake: 10 mg for adults. If you are taking over 300 mg, seek professional guidance.

Herbs

Herbs are as healing to the gums and teeth as they are for your total body. Herbal therapy for the gums is both preventive in nature and can also help you to reverse gum disease naturally.

- *To build gums:* cydonia, manihot, echinacea, and/or rosemary
- *To stop bleeding gums:* calendula, chlorophyll, and bone meal

- *To prevent inflammation and gingivitis:* echeveria, erodium, jatropha, krameria, morus, myrtus, nicotiana, oxalis, punica, paphanus, and/or sedum

Herbs rich in protein can help you prevent and reverse existing gum problems. These include dandelion, currant, parsley, and okra. Others are alfalfa, bee pollen, cloves, cumin, dill, fennel, and ginger.

Here are some ways you can incorporate these herbs into your diet:

Dandelion can be used as a tea. The roasted root (dandelion) and its extract are used as coffee substitutes or as an instant coffee.

Currant can be used as a flavoring in foods.

Parsley is used to reduce sulfur in the mouth. It is rich in protein. Putting some on the side of a plate looks attractive, and should be eaten at the end of a meal, since it freshens the breath.

Okra is a food that can be used in drinks and in a salad.

Alfalfa sprouts are used in salads and can be helpful in treating diabetics.

Bee pollen can be found in gel form, as an herbal tea gum, as well as in extract form.

Cloves, clove bud oil, and clove leaf oil are widely used in flavoring many food products.

Cumin is a major flavor component in herbal teas.

Dill is also used as a flavor component for food.

Fennel is found in teas, tinctures, or in honey syrup.

Ginger is used as a domestic spice.

Oregano is a flavor ingredient for foods.

You can replace your coffee with teas made from these ingredients. Herbal teas will help reverse your gum disease and soothe the digestive system. Coffee (even decaffeinated) is reported to stimulate gastric secretions that can have harmful effects on the gum tissue. (If you must drink coffee, please add cream to neutralize the acids.)

Protein

Protein forms the collagen-woven framework that gets mineralized into bone formation. Foods rich in protein include dandelion, currant, milk, parsley, okra, meat, fish, cheese, and legumes.

Recommended daily intake: 20 to 80 grams.

Getting Motivated to Eat Healthy

Even now that we know what foods and vitamins to eat to keep us and our gums healthy, we need to understand *how* to keep motivated to eat healthily. It is not easy to turn away from junk food. There is an instant reward that takes place when people eat fast food. We must use self-control to direct ourselves toward eating properly.

What was once the diet of the past is now becoming the diet of the future—one that will keep us healthy. The ancients ate only living food that was naturally grown. What is living food? It is any food that is not processed by heat, freezing, canning, drying, pickling, or sweetening. It is grown without sprays or chemicals. It is any food that promotes good health by protecting all the vitamins, minerals, enzymes, and trace elements that give the body its energy, power, and resistance to infection, strain, and stress. This is the type of food you should be seeking to keep your mouth healthy.

Start off by trying to eat one raw meal, one fruit meal, and one hot meal (freshly prepared) each day. Eat only when hungry, and *never* overeat. Do not eat when you are tired or emotionally upset. Also avoid combining many different types of food at one meal. Avoid overcooked vegetables and burned, processed, synthetically bleached, or refined foods. Avoid artificial flavors, imitation fruit, and imitation dairy products.

You will find miso soup and herbal teas especially soothing to the gum tissue. Herbs incorporated in a tea bag soothe the tissue directly. Look to pages 133–135 and 137 for which herbs to choose. At the Tooth Spa I offer my patients green tea and herbal teas, including echinacea tea and one made with a mixture of fine imported herbs. I find that these teas assist in healing after a gum treatment. I instruct my patients to have miso soup or a light meal after a gum treatment.

Here are some of my recommendations for people who wish to eat a healthier diet but like to snack during the day. Choose to snack on pilaf, miso soup (never boil miso soup), sprouts, alfalfa sprouts, lentils, sunflower seeds, buckwheat greens, roasted nuts, or popcorn. Note: Popcorn may be a healthy snack, but the shells of the popcorn can easily slide under the gum. Use an oral irrigator to dislodge the shells if this happens.

Other herbs that heal gums and are used in the prevention and reversal of gum disease include:

Arnica: found in beverages, baked goods, gelatins, and herbal extracts

Rosemary: found in oils, teas, and as an ingredient for food flavoring. Has antimicrobial properties.

Stevia: a natural sweetener. Found in foods, and can be added for a sweet flavor to teas or if you need to drink coffee.

Honey: a natural sweetener

Myrrh: found in extracts

Tea tree oil: found in oils and extracts

Lavender: found in oils. Flowers and oils are used as flavoring in tea and foods.

Macrobiotics

I would like to share with you a diet that is five thousand years old, and from the Orient. This specific diet helps build vitality, nerves, and muscular strength. The mouth, which is in direct relationship to the body, reacts accordingly, thereby giving the gums and teeth added vitality and strength. The art of macrobiotics helps in the understanding of longevity, the wholesome, creative life, and the balancing of yin and yang (passive and active) elements that exist in everything and every activity—not just food. It emphasizes harmony with nature, especially through following a diet that consists mostly of whole grains, beans, vegetables, and moderate amounts of seafood and fruit.

How does one achieve the yin-yang balance that is so important to a macrobiotic diet? In food, for example, meat, fish, and poultry are a yang group. The proportion of yin to yang that should be attained in a healthy person is five to one—five yin foods to one yang food. The following is a classification of yin and yang food groups. Simply select five food choices from a yin group, and one from a yang group.

Vegetables (yin): eggplant, tomato, sweet potato, potato, pimento, green beans, cucumbers, asparagus, spinach, artichoke, bamboo shoots, mushrooms, green pea, celery, purple cabbage, beet, white cabbage, dandelion, lettuce, endive, kale, radish, garlic, onion, parsley, pumpkin, winter squash, carrots, burdock, watercress, seaweed, and agar

Legumes (yin): soy beans, green beans, white beans, split peas, kidney beans, pinto beans, lentils, chickpeas, black beans, and aduki beans

Sweets (yin): sugar, honey, molasses, rice syrup, barley malt syrup

Oils (yin): soy oil, coconut oil, peanut oil, corn oil, margarine, olive oil, sunflower oil, sesame oil, and safflower oil

Fruit (yin): pineapple, grapefruit, lime, orange, lemon, tangerine, grapes, papaya, mango, dates, prunes, avocado, cantaloupe, banana, fig, pear, peach, apricot, blueberry, blackberry, watermelon, olive, strawberry, cherry, and apple

Seeds (yin): sunflower, pumpkin, squash, and sesame

Dairy (yin): ice cream, yogurt, sour cream, sweet cream, butter, cow's milk, cheese, goat's milk, and goat cheese

Beverages (yin): tea, vinegar, mint, chamomile, coffee, fruit juice, champagne, wine, beer, mineral soda (carbonated), water (deep well), thyme, chicory, barley coffee, grain tea, dandelion coffee, and ginseng root

Nuts (yin): cashew, peanut, pistachio, pecan, almond, walnut, and chestnut

Animal food (yang): snails, frogs, pork, lamb, horse, rabbit, chicken, pigeon, partridge, beef, duck, turkey, egg, and pheasant

Seafood (yang): oysters, clams, octopus, eel, carp, mussel, halibut, lobster, trout, sole, crab, salmon, herring, sardine, shrimp, red snapper, and caviar

Condiments (yang): sauerkraut, gomasio, miso, tamari, tekka, and sea salt

PART III

PROFESSIONAL DENTAL HINTS

Part III is meant to increase your understanding of dental health, by adding confidence and expertise. Knowledge of your mouth can help you in reversing gum disease naturally. I will make suggestions, and help you chart success toward reversing gum disease naturally. You do not have to be a professional dental hygienist or dentist to work expertly on your mouth. Also, I will give you professional dental hints that will enable you to have better control in the dental office. Dental fears are usually related to lack of knowledge of a specific topic. In this part of the book, you will also learn how to find a dentist and hygienist whom you can trust. With all of this information, you will be on the road to reversing gum disease naturally, and professionally.

The next chapter will help you become a "lay professional." You will learn how to chart the mouth and note the differences and changes in your mouth.

8

Charting Success for the Reversal of Gum Disease

In most dental offices, charting the mouth helps a professional review notes to prepare a treatment plan. I will help to direct you in charting your mouth successfully. The diagrams of your mouth that result will help you chart your rate of success as a "lay professional" in dental hygiene.

Note: A chart should be made at your first exam by your dental professional. Ask him or her for a copy of your chart. There are two types of charts: one is an overview of your mouth, while the other diagrams the pocket depth of your gums. It would be good to have both.

Charting and Drawing an Outline of Your Mouth

View your mouth in a well-lit room with a mirror. If you have a dental mirror, use it to look at the inside of your mouth.

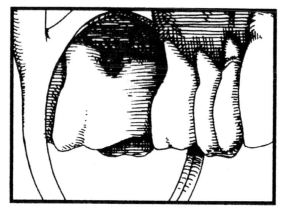

Using a mouth mirror.

If you do not have a dental mouth mirror, then go to your nearest drug store and order one. If you are having trouble locating one, feel free to call me (my number is listed at the end of the book).

Looking at your teeth as a "lay professional" may be a new experience for you. Take the small mouth mirror and insert it into your mouth to reflect your back teeth. (Again, make sure the room is well lit.) View your teeth through the mouth mirror. Your teeth may not be as perfectly lined up as you thought. Check to see if you have all your molars. There should be twelve molars, including the wisdom teeth. Most people do not have room for their wisdom teeth. See where your gum line meets your teeth.

Now, get a notepad and keep all your dental notes in this book. After you have viewed your teeth with a mouth mirror, you will use the notebook to chart your teeth. Here's how you should start:

1. On the first page, write the motto "Save Your Smile."
   Date each page and make notations about your teeth.
2. On the second page, write the name of your dentist,
   his or her phone number and address, and the name
   of your dental hygienist.
3. After recording this information, write down the
   date of your last dental appointment, and then write
   down the date of your next appointment or the
   approximate date you are due for a repeat visit.
4. Next, take a clean piece of paper and start charting
   your teeth.

Right   **Left**

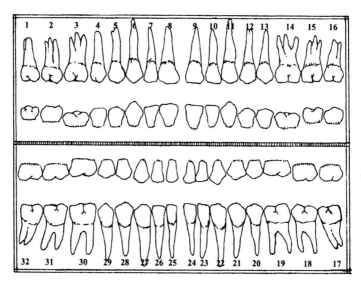

A dental chart used in a dental office.

5. On a side column list any spaces where teeth are missing. Try to evaluate how many teeth have been removed from these spaces.

6. Next, mark down the silver or white fillings that you can see, differentiating between both. To do this, place your mouth mirror around your teeth, then look at the chart and draw the outline of each filling on the chart. (You may want to photocopy the chart and mark up the photocopy instead.) Note that "Right" means teeth on the *right* side of your mouth and "Left" means the *left* side. For example, your lower right second molar is tooth #31. If this molar has a large surface filling, then take a pencil and make the same shape filling on tooth #31 on the left side of your dental chart. After you outline the shape of the filling on the chart, pencil it in if it is silver, but do not fill it in if it is a white filling. This shows the difference between a silver filling and a white filling. It is important to differentiate between the two.

7. Elsewhere on the paper, mark any abnormalities that you may see on your cheeks or on the top of your tongue.

8. Also write down the color of your gums (e.g., pale/pink, pink, deep magenta). For example, if your gums are deep magenta around your upper front teeth, mark this down and try to specify which tooth or teeth. Write it like this: "magenta deep purple on upper right central tooth."

9. Look at your gum line and try to draw what you see on paper. When a tooth looks long, it is most likely

due to recession or excessive shrinkage of your gums. If you see areas that seem to be loose and stretchy, then mark the tooth numbers down and write "loose and stretchy." If you have areas with a receded gum line, then mark "gum recession" next to the tooth number. If the gums look like they are receding in a certain area, draw a line above the tooth area and write "receded gum area around upper right tooth #3."

10. If your gums look puffy and irritated, mark down the tooth as best as you can (e.g., "tooth #4 has gum inflammation").

11. Now floss your teeth, and if any areas are bleeding due to your flossing, mark down the approximate tooth or area. Smell the floss after flossing. If it has a harsh smell, then you may have excessive bacteria in that area. Mark the corresponding tooth on the chart. If your gums seem to be bleeding, even when you are not brushing and massaging them, chart this information as well. It is important to date all the information, especially when unusual conditions arise.

12. Mark down any crowns and bridges on your chart. A crown should look only slightly different from your natural tooth, and sometimes shows a line near the gum line. If the crown is made of gold, however, it is obviously easy to differentiate from your own tooth. Let's say you have a crown on your upper right second molar. You would circle tooth #7 on the left side of the dental chart with blue ink. If you have a crown and bridge, it is very probable that your gums are

loose and spongy in that area. Most crowns have a slight edge, and the gum tissue gets loose and stretchy around these restorations. If the gum bleeds in certain areas, look carefully and mark down the restoration that is sitting near that gum area. Bridges hold food and bacteria and usually create irritations because they are difficult to clean. If you have large silver or white fillings, it is also most probable that the gums are loose around these teeth.

13. If you believe that a tooth has a laminate on it, circle it on the chart and label it a laminate. To differentiate a laminate from a crown, look at the front and back of the tooth with your dental mouth mirror. If the back of your tooth looks like your natural tooth and the front looks shiny, then it is most likely a laminate.

14. An implant is a false tooth that screws into the jawbone. It replaces an entire tooth. If you remember what tooth is an implant, mark this on the chart.

15. If you have a partial denture (a denture that attaches to your existing teeth), chart it by drawing teeth in the place of the missing teeth with a blue pen. If you have a denture, mark the "missing teeth" and then make a circle where the denture is replacing your own teeth.

16. Make additional notes about abnormalities, such as teeth that seem to be loose. Note those areas where teeth seem to be loose. If a tooth is on its side or slightly bending, make note of this. If teeth seem to be discolored, mark this down over the tooth number.

17. Note teeth that are higher or lower than the other teeth surrounding them. Teeth can extrude or recede if they are not opposed by another tooth. Gravity

will move these teeth out of position. This happens if only one of your wisdom teeth is pulled.

18. Don't forget to chart the inside of your teeth. The gum line on the inside of your teeth is equally as important as the gum line on the outside. Look at the chart and you will notice that your teeth have a front and inside view. Draw the outside gum line and then draw the inside gum line in red ink.

You have just completed your first chart.

Once You've Made Your First Chart

You should refer to your dental notebook every month. Remember to mark the date each time. Compare your mouth to how it was depicted on the chart before. Look carefully at your gum line.

Mark the color of your gums, and note if there have been any changes. See if you find any improvements. Check the gum line from before to see if any of the areas that looked irregular are better.

Looking at your most recent chart, chart a comparison view of your gum line. Using a green-ink pen or pencil, trace your gums. Note the differences from your last chart to this chart. Take a mouth mirror and try to get a good look and make a line on the chart that most resembles the appearance of your gum line. Follow this till you complete the review of your whole mouth.

Look closely at your teeth, and then take the back of your mouth mirror and touch each tooth, to see if any of them move. You can also do this with the back of an ordinary toothbrush. If you see that some of your teeth are moving, then note this on the chart. Most teeth naturally have some slight movement, but if the movement of the tooth is excessive, then note this on the chart.

Make notes about any tartar buildup. If you can clearly see tartar on the inside of the lower teeth by using a mouth mirror, then note this on the chart. If the tartar buildup looks lighter, then note this on the chart.

If you feel your mouth is a lot healthier than it was before, then put a gold star next to the notes. This will make you feel good, and you can immediately make comparisons toward the reversal of gum disease naturally.

Under "notes," also mark and date any change in your diet.

This comparison of your charts will educate you as to how you are improving. If you see little improvement, then your at-home treatment should be looked at and changed. Bring your notes to your dentist or hygienist and ask for assistance.

A Healthy Mouth

A healthy mouth has a light, happy appearance; it speaks of joy, youth, and contentment. The mouth should be free from pain and disease. The appearance of your mouth in a healthier state should also be charted and noted. As mentioned before, chart the color and tone of the tissue (e.g., pink = tight tissue). If you feel your gums are in better condition, then date the chart and mark the improvements. You can then review this chart in a month.

9

Setting Up an At-Home Hygiene Center
The Tooth Spa Program

Professionally speaking, you have arrived! The next step is to create a dental hygiene home care station in your bathroom. Following these directions, you will have an ideal dental hygiene home care station.

Think of your bathroom area as a small professional workstation and use your mouth chart (see chapter 8) as a reference point. The chart will give you added professional information needed to work clearly and visually on your gum line. Look at the areas that you have marked that may need more work. Concentrate on those areas.

An At-Home Spa Approach to Dental Hygiene

Look at your bathroom and evaluate where you can set up your equipment. If you have a small bathroom with little room on the sink, then buy a shelf to store your appliances and products. The items you will need are:

- Toothbrushes, electric and manual
- Floss
- Oral irrigator
- Herbal extracts
- Sea salt
- Baking soda (sodium bicarbonate)
- Rubber-tipped stimulators
- Mouth mirror
- Toothpaste—herbal and baking soda

Make sure the room is well lit. Your mouth is dark, and if the room is also dark, you will have a hard time viewing your mouth.

The Tooth Spa Hygiene Station

The "tooth spa" program is an innovative gum-care program adapted from treatments I had at a spa I frequented in New York. Dental hygiene professionals and specialists are so concerned with the removal of tartar and bacteria they often omit the healing necessities of the gums. I developed the "tooth spa" program because people are able to understand the need to clean and massage their gums by associating gum care with skin care.

An at-home spa approach to dental hygiene home care will allow you to enjoy your home care treatments. The spa approach is a softer and gentler approach compared to conventional scientific methods. What makes a person excited about going to a spa? Perhaps the decor of the room, the aroma, the music, and the soft massage treatments. You too can make your bathroom into a spa facility for your teeth and gums and, most important, create an added healing effect toward reversing gum disease naturally.

Light a scented candle and place it near your dental hygiene products. The healing scent of the candle will add therapeutic energy to the treatments. Play soft, meditative music.

Now visualize your mouth surrounded with white healing light, then visualize a purple light surrounding the white light. Direct these healing images toward the gum line. You will be ready to heal and soothe the gum tissue.

The parts of the "spa" treatment we'll cover include:

- Brush and toned massage
- The tooth wrap
- Whirlpool cleansing
- Intercleansing massage
- Final brush and tone
- The all-over glow

However, in order to embark on this program, you must first get the necessary equipment.

Brush and Toned Massage

The soft massage and cleansing approach is similar to the spa approach for the total body. Think of your gum tissue as you would the skin on your face. Use a massage tool (a toothbrush) for the gums. You should have a manual and an electric toothbrush available. I suggest choosing a special soft bristle brush designed for gum care.

Take the side of the brush and direct it to the gums. Then shimmy the brush back and forth using your own healing energy. I say "healing energy" because we *all* have healing energy (see chapter 6). I had a nurse in and she thanked me for helping her "connect" with her mouth. She said that the mouth was a mystery to her and she was afraid of hurting herself. If you see blood on the brush, do not fear. The tissue might be loose and spongy, and brushing with a gentle massage will help the circulation of the gum tissue. Good circulation brings healing cells to the surface to tighten and strengthen the gum tissue. If your gums are loose and spongy, then food and bacteria can lodge under the gum, causing loose irritated tissue. You therefore must cleanse and massage the gum tissue.

A Word on Toothbrushes

It is important to learn to use a manual toothbrush, which provides you with great control. I have watched many people merely brush their teeth, and thus miss the important performance of gum massage.

The more innovative products that help with the massage of the gums are electric toothbrushes. These brushes come in all sizes and shapes. The beauty of such a brush with a little round head is that it moves in a circular motion, and can focus on each individual gum around the tooth. It is small enough that it helps in controlling your focus on what you are doing. As for sonic brushes, they operate at a higher vibration and may irritate the gums if used incorrectly.

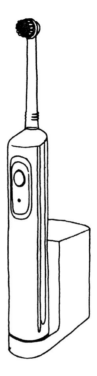

Round-bristle electric brush.

Therefore, get professional instruction first before using any electric oral hygiene product.

Massage of the gums should be done first and last during our spa dental hygiene program.

The Tooth Wrap

Have you ever been to a spa and had a body wrap? You can detoxify with this procedure. Heated towels that have been dipped in herbs are wrapped around your body, and the herb essences are absorbed into the body via the pores of your skin. A seaweed wrap is similar—the body is wrapped with seaweed, then covered with heated towels and wrapped in plastic. Then you are covered with a blanket. This allows the nutrients from the seaweed to be absorbed through the skin into the body. It is also very relaxing; you might even fall into a deep meditation.

Now your teeth and gums can get the same kind of spa treatment with a "tooth wrap," designed so that herbal products can be absorbed into the gums. The new cells of the gum tissue need to be nurtured and kept vital, while the old tissue is removed. Herbal toothpaste can help detoxify the mouth, especially with acid breath due to eating excessive amounts of sugars. Take two 2"-by-2" pieces of gauze and place a dot of Bioforce's herbal toothpaste on each piece. Then open the gauze. Notice that most of the water in the paste has been absorbed by the gauze, leaving the substance thicker than normal. Using the gauze as an applicator, spread the toothpaste on the gums. Now remove the gauze, leaving a thickened herbal paste on the gums, and floss the toothpaste under the gums. Then wrap the floss with the herbal paste just under the gum cuff. Finally, massage the herbal paste into the tissue to nurture the cells and give the gums strength.

Whirlpool Cleansing

Most spas have a whirlpool to sit in, which helps your circulatory system and enables you to relax. What would a whirlpool cleansing do for the mouth? Such a cleansing rewards the mouth for the work it does—grinding and ripping the foods that you eat. You can do this by using an oral irrigator, which not only makes your mouth feel fresh but also invigorates the gum tissue and cleans under the gum cuff.

Use an oral irrigator (such as a Water Pik) with two capfuls of peroxyl or peroxide added to the water, then alternate with a natural mouth rinse. Cleansing of the gum cuff should be done daily, preferably in the morning and evening. The hydrogen peroxide helps reduce the anaerobic bacteria (bacteria that live without oxygen, which eat the bone). Be careful, however: Peroxide can be caustic if it is used too much, and so you should alternate it with an herbal mouthwash.

The temperature in the oral irrigator should be tepid, not too hot or too cold. Fill the container and then use the hose apparatus aimed at gum line at a right angle. Do not use too high a pressure. The whirlpool helps to dislodge the food and bacteria from under the gum and also helps reduce anaerobic bacteria.

This kind of cleansing is as important as a massage. You must cleanse under the gum cuff to have vital healthy tissue. This will keep your gum tissue attached and healthy next to your teeth.

Intercleansing Massage

Cleansing in-between your teeth is important, because this is where food and bacteria like to hide. Floss is an adjunct in interproximal cleansing, and must be used correctly. Do not snap the floss, as it can cut the gum tissue. If you have a tight contact between teeth, do not force the floss. It will cut into the gum tissue, which can lead to infection and abscesses. (See chapter 6 for tips on flossing correctly.)

Another method of interproximal cleansing is to use an orangewood stick (see chapter 6). An orangewood stick is similar to a toothpick, but is softer and can be used to massage between your teeth.

Or you can choose to use a fine interproximal brush. This brush will open the tissue, allowing you to push food particles out. Please only use a fine interproximal brush, even if the space between the teeth is large. I find that if you do not use a fine brush, the tissue can be stretched and loosened, causing much damage.

Next, use a rubber tip to help to reduce the swelling of gum tissue. It can remove plaque and some food around the gum cuff. Used properly, it can offer stimulation and circulation to the gum tissue. Outline your teeth with the rubber tip, and when you are in-between the teeth (in the interproximal areas), use the thicker part of the tip to massage the tissue. Work around each tooth with rhythm and make a circle when you get between the teeth. Using rhythm will make this less tiring.

Final Brush and Tone

Using rhythm, floss first, oral irrigate, brush and tone, and feel the healing energy therapeutically go into the gums. Healing rhythms are essential for oral hygiene. Play some music as you work the gums. Divide your mouth into four sections. Begin with the upper right and lower right, followed by the upper left and lower left. Using a soft brush and herbal toothpaste, work the brush at the gum line with rhythm. Feel the massage as you shimmy the brush from side to side.

The All-Over Glow

Using a small dental mirror, check the glow and health of your teeth and gums. Take the dental mirror and place it at the back of your teeth, then look into a larger mirror. See your gums and teeth and how you have helped revitalize the tissue. Gum care can be vital to your health—and a healthy smile is a confident smile.

You have used the softer spa approach to dental hygiene home care. If you look forward to treating your gums and teeth, then you will work methodically and readily every day on hygiene home care. This can save you thousands of dollars in the long run.

Creating Good Habits and Finding the Motivation

Having fun with oral hygiene can be accomplished with this softer spa approach. Learning to love your teeth and smile is important. Self-love can be represented in your smile. And why shouldn't you smile with confidence?

It is important to create good habits in oral hygiene. To motivate yourself to try and keep to this at-home spa approach, put a note on your mirror that daily care will save you many thousands of dollars in a lifetime.

Don't forget to set the stage. Light a lavender-scented candle before you begin, or get a spray of lavender. Be positive! Do not resent working on your health. Your mouth can keep you *young*. Aging takes place when our parts start breaking down. Have you ever noticed an elderly person with natural, healthy looking teeth? This can be you!

Working with rhythm, as discussed, will help make the time pass by quickly. Once you develop the habit, it can become second nature for you. Setting the stage for an at-home dental hygiene health station can be fun and invigorating.

Plus, waking up in the morning to an invigorating session of dental hygiene will help to stimulate your mind. Think of how you feel when your mouth is dry and smelly. Are you prepared to face the day with positive energy feeling like this? Your mouth should be feeling light and healthy, not heavy and dull. Stimulating the gum tissue will also stimulate your mental state. Clean, fresh breath will help you start the day right.

The evening is also an important time for dental hygiene. Using the proper tools in the evening for your gums and teeth will reduce the bacteria likely to invade your gums and teeth at night due to diminished saliva. You will rest better, knowing that you have removed many of the bacterial bugs that are waiting to invade your teeth and gums while you are asleep.

10

Finding the Right Professional to Guide You in the Natural Reversal of Gum Disease

How to Find the Right Professional for the Care of Your Gums and Teeth

You have just taken an important step in becoming a "lay professional" in dental hygiene at home. As an educated patient, you now have the opportunity to find a compatible dental professional with whom to work.

First, try to communicate with your present dentist and hygienist. If they are happy to answer questions and offer you additional information on dental health, then you are with the right dental professionals.

However, if they seem bothered by your questions and do not want to work with you, it is imperative that you find a dental professional who will. You will want to try to locate a holistic and caring professional. The word "holistic" is a direct reference to mind, body, and spirit, and to connecting the body parts and seeing the person as a whole. I have been called a "holistic hygienist," not only because I use herbs during my treatment but also because I treat the patient as a whole. I may see an obese patient and try to help motivate that patient to self-care in hygiene and diet. Caring leads you, as a professional, to a direct action of holistic care.

If you need a new dental professional, it is important to do some research, and there are different areas to explore.

Yellow Pages

If you open the Yellow Pages in your area, you will see many dental professionals listed. How can you find the right professional from the Yellow Pages? Read the ads! What does the ad say? Is the dental professional marketing his practice to fit your needs? You might see such words as "caring," "gentle," "holistic," "nonsurgical gum programs," "discounted dentistry," "free exam," and more. It is important to read beyond the words and discover the truth about the dental professional. After reading the ad, call the office. If the person who answers the phone seems friendly and is equipped to answer your questions, then you may have reached the right office. If you are turned off by the person who answers the phone, it is still possible that the dental professional is good, but less likely. Before calling the office, however, have your questions on hand and ask those that are important to you. Here are some suggestions:

- Does the dental professional work as a holistic practitioner? If not, what methods does he or she use?
- Does he or she have a nonsurgical approach to gum disease?

- Does the office work with patients on a payment plan?
- Can the office accept my insurance?
- Is the dental professional available for emergencies?
- Can I have references and speak with other patients who are pleased with the office? (optional)
- What university did the dental professional graduate from?
- How much expertise does the dental professional have?
- Does the dental office have the latest equipment?
- What sterilization procedures does the office have?

Many of these questions might not be answered in the first phone call. However, if some of the questions are answered to your liking, then make a consultation appointment at the office. At the office you will be able to get more questions answered.

At that appointment, look around to see how neat and clean the office is. Ask to see the sterilization area and techniques used. Remember, they need you as a patient or they would not be advertising. Do not be afraid to be inquisitive, you are looking for a quality professional who has patience to work with you on this level.

A concern should also be that the dentist and dental hygienist have a good working relationship. They both should be happy and love their work.

Word-of-Mouth Referral Sources

Finding a competent, knowledgeable, professional, and affordable dentist and dental hygienist can be a difficult task. Most people base their search essentially on word of mouth. However, someone else's idea of a good dentist is often subjective. So how can word-of-mouth suggestions work for you? Ask the person who is offering the referral some of these questions:

- Is the dental professional holistic in approach? Does he or she have a nonsurgical approach to gum disease?
- Does the dental professional work with a light touch?
- Does the dental professional work with empathy?
- Is the office clean and neat?
- What kind of sterilization methods are used?
- Does the office work with a payment plan?
- Does the office accept credit cards?
- Will the office accept my insurance?
- Why do you specifically like this office?
- Can you compare this dental office to your last office and then tell me why you prefer this office?
- Do you look forward to seeing your dental professional? Why?
- Are you satisfied when you leave the office?
- Have you had fewer problems with your teeth and gums since you have begun going to this office?

After many of your questions have been answered to your satisfaction, you are ready to call for an appointment. When making an appointment, you should mention your referral source to the receptionist. A referral is regarded highly by a dental practice. There is no greater compliment to the office and the professional than getting word-of-mouth referrals.

Web Sites

Many dental practices are now on the Web. You can view my Web site at toothfairyshow.com, which will introduce you to the office. If certain procedures are used and you are interested in these procedures, you can view the information on the Web site. Most Web sites can be categorized as "Holistic Dentistry," "Gum Disease Prevention," and "Cosmetic Dentistry." You can try various search engines and select the category you are most interested in.

Many Web sites have photos of the professional, and you can see if the image of the person is the image you want. Seeing a face is worth a thousand words.

Questions can be directed to these Web sites. Some Web sites, including my own, have e-mail addresses. You can e-mail your questions on the Internet. It is important to know that many offices are very busy, and the opportunity to answer your questions about a practice may be limited.

Suggested questions to ask on the Web:

- Are you holistic in your practice?
- What materials do you use?
- How much do you charge for a consultation and dental work?
- Where are you located?
- Are you caring and gentle?
- How many people do you employ?
- Do you work on patients yourself?
- What are your credentials?
- What sterilization methods do you employ?

Media: Radio and Television Referral Sources

Another way to search for a dental professional is through the media. Periodically you hear about a dental professional who has a radio or television show. Being able to listen to the person speak or just watch a dental professional on television can be one advantage over print advertising and even word-of-mouth referrals.

Listening to someone on the radio will help you consider how this person presents himself or herself. Presentation is very important professionally! If a professional takes the time to appear on radio or television, then he or she might have a higher interest in educating the public in dental health and be more in tune with your needs.

Dial 1-800-Dentist

You can find 1-800-Dentist advertisements on television commercials. The dentists listed pay for the advertisements and their listings on 1-800-Dentist.

Magazine Articles

Be cautious. Many people hire public relations professionals to help them market their services. So be careful of magazine articles that name celebrity clients in the article, as this doesn't necessarily mean the dentist is of the highest quality. Read between the lines.

Finding the Right Dental Hygienist

You might like the dentist you have chosen, but might end up with a dental hygienist who works in the office but who does not fill your needs. If the dental hygienist who works for your dentist doesn't satisfy your needs, then use the dentist of your choice, but select your own dental hygienist. If you are unhappy with your hygienist, you can still ask your dentist to work on you while you use an independent contractor dental hygienist. She or he must be authorized by the dentist she or he rents a chair from. If you need a referral source, my number and address are listed in this book. I can refer readers to other hygienists who are independent contractors throughout the United States.

Select a holistic dental hygienist, one who works with natural products and herbs. He or she works on the whole person and uses many systems and plans, including diet and nutritional control.

Questions to ask to find a good dental hygienist professional include:

- What is your philosophy as a dental hygienist?
- How many years have you practiced?
- Do you love your work?
- Do you believe in the nonsurgical approach to periodontal disease?
- Are you empathetic?
- Are you light-handed?
- Do you teach dental hygiene home care?

A dental hygienist can prevent the onset of periodontal disease, and if the disease has already progressed, he or she may help reverse the disease process.

Here are some of the questions that you should ask your new dental professional on the first visit for treatment for a nonsurgical approach to gum disease:

- How deep are my gum pockets? (Gum pockets, the spaces between the gum and the bone, are measured by the hygienist to determine the severity of your gum disease.)
- Do you think you can help reverse my gum disease?
- What is your natural approach for reversal of my condition?
- Do your treatments hurt? What should I expect during treatment?
- Is there pain after the treatment?
- Will you help me put together a dental hygiene home care program?
- How many treatments will I need?
- How many times a year will I have to see you?
- What is the cost of these treatments?
- Have you had good results from a nonsurgical approach to gum disease?
- Can gum disease return after treatment?
- Do you work with any specific diet?
- Should I stay away from any food during treatment?
- Should I take Advil or aspirin during or before treatment?
- How does helping remove gum disease help in total wellness?
- Will I be able to see the results?

Ask these questions before and after treatment if necessary. Answers to your questions will help you heal! Educational information removes questions from the mind, leaving you secure and confident to heal! Trust and confidence can be achieved with knowledge, which will then reinforce the professional treatments.

Here are some hints on how to work closely and more efficiently with your dental professional:

- Be on time for your appointment.
- Try not to cancel or change too many appointments.
- If you have a medical or physical problem, be sure to inform your dental professional.
- Don't squirm or fall off the chair. (Trust!)
- Don't rush the professional. Asking your dental professional to hurry up may hinder your treatment.
- Do not try to compromise the dental professional's fees. If you cannot afford the fees, say so in the beginning. Do not manipulate the dental professional to accept less than his or her standard fee. Payment plans can be presented before treatment starts.
- Do not eat candy or chew gum before a treatment.
- If you are not sure about the treatment, then ask questions before it starts.
- Compliment the hygienist who is working on you. Don't forget, he or she has been working hard all day trying to save teeth.
- Schedule another appointment when you leave.
- Pay for your treatment promptly if possible. Don't wait for the office to bill you.
- Go for your follow-up visits routinely, and schedule your maintenance visits ahead of time.

These rules will help you develop a better relationship with your dental professional. He or she will value your consideration. It is important that an empathetic connection is made between the dental professional and the patient. Pretend that you are the dental professional and evaluate what your needs would be to care for you as the patient. This could help you to understand the dental professional's needs. Empathize!

How to Work with a Conventional Dental Practitioner in Natural Healing

Not all dentists employ or are natural healers themselves. It is more the norm to have a dentist work in a conventional style. If you have selected a conventional dentist and still wish to use his or her services, then I would suggest that you locate a holistic dental hygienist in addition to help you reverse gum disease naturally.

However, if you prefer a nonsurgical approach, you must let your dentist know. If he or she objects, then you have to decide if you are working with the right professional.

11

For Parents

Your Role in Preventing Gum Disease in Children

If you set a good example in dental hygiene home care, your child will be motivated to save his or her teeth. Become a good example for your children, and you will motivate them. Don't wait for disaster to strike. *Now* is the time you can help your child to become motivated in keeping his or her teeth.

All about Germs

The mouth holds thousands of germs, and these germs can spread throughout the body. So make sure that your child replaces his or her toothbrush frequently. If it is an electric toothbrush, then replace the head of the toothbrush frequently. And make sure that he or she rinses the brush head in hot water to remove the germs.

What can motivate children is to tell them about germs. Remind children that germs can spread from not taking care of their teeth. Tooth brushing, and brushing the top of the tongue, will help in removing the bacteria from the mouth. This will inhibit the germs from spreading throughout the body. Also, talk with your children and tell them that sugar turns to acid, and therefore all sweets contain acids that eat away at their teeth. If this occurs, they will have to have this decay removed with a drill and filled. Do not scare the child—motivate him or her. Sit down and openly talk about tooth brushing, and how this can brush away the acid from the sugar. Also discuss how tooth brushing can prevent decay. A few minutes a day will keep your child's teeth healthy. Pick up a small plastic two-minute hourglass, and tell your child to brush his teeth for as long as it takes the hourglass to empty. This makes brushing fun!

Teaching Your Child about Gum Massage

It's easy to prevent gum disease in children, and they have a better cleansing saliva than adults. The saliva is thinner and less acidic, which lessens plaque formation. Still, proper massage of the gums at an early age is important. You can help your children to find their gum line (where the teeth meet the gums). While children rarely get gum disease, they can become candidates for future gum disease if they do not massage their gums effectively. Massaging the gums will lead to healthy tissue.

Have your child look at your mouth, and show him or her where your gum line is. Then work with your child to show him how the massage of the gums feels. It's important for children to learn how much pressure to exert on the gum. This process should be followed after tooth brushing. An electric toothbrush might better enable your child to learn the rhythm of the brush style.

Follow these two steps as if playing "show and tell":

1. First work on your child with the manual toothbrush, on the teeth and gums. Do not forget the gums, even on a young child. Make little circles starting on the gums to bring circulation to the tissue.
2. Use an electric toothbrush to massage the gums. It is motivating to have the child use an electric brush, and brushing can be done in a fun and playful manner.

If you help your child in show and tell, he or she will understand the exact pressure needed to cleanse and massage their gums. Watch him do it the next time. Children will gain confidence if you show them correctly. Use a gentle massage action on the gums. If your child is using an electric brush, work gently around and on the gum tissue.

When Your Child Has Braces

A child with braces might be a candidate for gingivitis, with possible surgery needed after the removal of the braces.

When braces are worn, gum tissue can swell and stretch. The tooth movement causes pressure on the gum and this creates stretching of the gum fibers and causes irritation. You may notice blood on your child's toothbrush. If so, make sure that your child massages his or her gums daily with a natural cleansing toothpaste with baking soda.

Also, children who wear braces usually keep their mouths open at night. If this is what your child is doing, then use a natural aloe gel on his or her gums, or moisturize the gums at bedtime with Vaseline.

Breaking the Thumb-Sucking Habit

Thumb sucking can be a cause of gum problems in children. There are germs on your childrens' fingers, and with thumb sucking they are constantly transmitting these germs into their mouths. The germs will be transferred to the soft gum tissue and the teeth. The gum tissue will get inflamed, leaving a red line or marginal gingivitis.

Thumb sucking is also bad because it can push the teeth out of alignment, and in one's adult years this can cause gum disease. The malaligned teeth become food traps, and the tissue can get irritated from food and bacteria that lie under the gum. So try to help break your child's habit at a young age.

Children who suck their thumbs are usually very independent and can be stubborn as well. This feeling of independence will help them as adults, but their stubbornness may make it more difficult to get them to stop the habit.

Strategies to stop thumb-sucking in children:

- Be patient with your child. He or she feels comfortable sucking his or her thumb.
- There are dental appliances that can be placed in the mouth to break the thumb-sucking habit. Consult a dentist.
- Use psychology and gently approach your child with information that the thumb is dirty and can cause sore throats and other infections in the body.

- Tell your child softly and with a nurturing attitude that the teeth will come forward (protrude) if he or she continues to suck his or her thumb.
- Thumb sucking is self-nurturing; try to nurture your child away from this habit.

Don't worry if the habit persists—most children break the habit when they are ready.

Motivating Your Child

It often seems that boys tend to be lazy when it comes to hygienic habits, and girls are a little more fastidious. Grimy teeth may seem more attractive to some boys—it makes them feel tough and masculine—while some girls are more detailed and punctilious with hygiene habits.

If you are the parent of a boy, then make sure he understands the need to prevent problems, and that if he does not clean his teeth, then the tops of the teeth can develop holes, which will lead to pain! Or try this strategy: I explain that your mouth is an energy field. If you keep your teeth clean and breathe well, then you will have more strength and energy to win games like baseball. This strategy seems to work in motivating boys to take better care of their teeth and gums. Fortunately, boys and young men today seem more concerned with appearance and presentation, and this will help in dental hygiene motivation.

If you have a daughter, you are at an advantage. Most girls, with the exception, perhaps, of tomboys, want to look pretty and clean. They can become highly motivated by talking about fresh, clean breath. Tell them that if they use a natural mouthwash, their breath will stay sweet.

Another way to get children, both boys and girls, motivated to keep their gums clean is to make sure you have the right dental products on hand. These include:

- *Soft toothbrushes:* If your child uses a hard bristle brush, he or she can rip the gum tissue and become a candidate for ridged enamel. Ridged and indented enamel will leave permanent grooves on the teeth and cause sensitivity to heat and cold and to sweets.
- *Oral irrigators:* An oral irrigator is especially important for children with braces. He or she will have a hard time flossing and brushing because of the hardware in his or her mouth. An oral irrigator will help remove the food particles that lie between the teeth and sit under the gum.
- *Natural toothpaste:* Have your child brush with a natural toothpaste. Most commercial toothpastes have a poison control warning on the box. (The warning is about excessive levels of fluoride. If fluoride is needed, then have your child use it as a rinse separate from tooth brushing.) Have your child start the day with a natural cleansing mint toothpaste, which can be invigorating. The best way to awaken with exuberance is to start by cleansing your mouth. Tell your child that healthy, sweet breath achieved through cleansing will bring a positive day.
- *Floss picks:* Such picks can be effective if your child has trouble flossing with just a piece of string floss.
- *Mouthwash:* Use a natural mouthwash. If your child's teeth are prone to decay, then a fluoride mouthwash might be necessary. (Fluoride is more important dur-

ing tooth development in pregnancy. If taken in prenatal vitamins, the developing teeth are mineralized.)

- *Electric toothbrushes:* If these products help motivate your child to brush, then buy them for him or her. Make sure that your child knows how to properly control the product. Do not let the product abrade the enamel or rip the gum tissue.

Putting Together a Child's At-Home Hygiene Station

The next thing you'll want to do is to set up a hygiene home care station for your child. This will keep your child motivated and focused. Here's how to design such a station:

- Make sure you have a well-lit area that's designated for your child.
- Put happy stickers with their favorite characters on their dental products. Line up all dental products together.
- Electric toothbrushes and oral irrigators can be fun and playful tools that will help motivate your child and keep their teeth and gums healthy.
- Make sure the mirror is clean and in a position that your child can look in it.
- Play music in the bathroom to add cheer to the day and create a calm, peaceful atmosphere before retiring.
- Use natural toothpaste. Children seem to prefer using a flavorful toothpaste, but it is more important to have healthful, natural products. Your child will discover these products are flavorful *and* healthful at the same time.

• Display photos of relatives, friends, and other children they know—even some child stars—who have healthy smiles.

Helpful Hints

As a parent concerned about your child's chances of gum disease, here are some things you should do:

• Routinely check your child's teeth.
• Reward your child occasionally for doing a good job in the prevention of dental disease.
• Try to limit sweets for your child.
• Set a good example for your child by working on your own teeth routinely in front of them.
• Tell your child how happy and clean your teeth are.
• Make going to the dentist a pleasant experience for you and your child.
• Do not project any of your own dental fears onto your child.
• Help to develop good oral hygiene habits by showing your child first how to work with dental tools.
• Flossing can be difficult for your child. Start by showing how you floss and brush.
• Massage your child's gums first so they will understand the right pressure on the gum tissue when they do it themselves.
• Smile often, and show your child the importance of healthy teeth.
• Make sure oral hygiene tools are kept clean. Routinely check the bristles of the toothbrush and make sure they

are not coated with food or dried toothpaste. This can cause problems for the teeth and gums. (Toothbrush bristles can hold germs, which can be then transmitted to your child.) You and your child can choose a soft bristle brush, but remember, it must be clean and fresh. The bristles should be smooth, and not worn.
- Use any "tooth fairy" money for fun but worthwhile products to help in saving one's teeth and gums.

Tips on Finding a Good Dental Professional for Your Child

It is important to find a good professional for your child. An early experience with a good professional can lead to a lifetime of healthy teeth and gums. Please follow the suggestions below to make this experience easier.

Many parents seem dumbfounded and ask neighbors or their pediatricians for recommendations—but do these people really know? A neighbor may be a good reference because of the experience his or her child had. Things to look for include:

- The office should be a cheerful and friendly place that will help reduce your child's fears.
- The office staff must be caring and personal.
- The dentist must have the personal time to answer your and your child's questions.
- The hygienist should be innovative and inspiring about hygiene home care lessons.
- Do not allow too many X rays, and make sure that you are aware of the treatment plan.

- If your child has decay on certain teeth, ask to see the X rays. If the dentist acts impatient about this request, then find another one!
- Ask for a fee schedule, so that there will not be any surprises thrown at you.

If the professional office you yourself visit sees children and you are confident in the staff, then use the office for your child. If you feel you would like a specialist (pedodontist), then remember you do not want an overly busy office that has little time for you and your child. Most children's dentists offices have a waiting room filled with toys. This can help relax your child—but it is more important that quality care be offered. Do your best to see that your child's happy and stress-free during visits. He or she should look forward to going to the dentist.

Systemic Diseases Affecting Early Onset of Periodontal Disease

It's important to know that some children may have systemic problems that affect the gum tissue. Juvenile diabetes affects the gums at an early age. Other systemic conditions affecting the periodontal condition of your child are associated with Down's syndrome (Mongolism). Papillon-Lefevre Syndrome (PLS) is a rare autosomal recessive genetic disease that is associated with prepubescent periodontitis. Your child can also develop prepubescent periodontitis, but this is rare. ANUG (acute necrotizing ulcerative gingivitis) is also a systemic condition that affects the onset of periodontal disease. ANUG has been observed as one of the oral symptoms of HIV and AIDS patients.

Steps to be taken if your child has any of these conditions:

- Have your child see a dentist/hygienist regularly.
- Oral care is important—explain that brushing, flossing, and oral irrigation are all musts.
- Make sure your child uses a toothpaste that is good for his or her total body health—ones with no harsh chemicals added and no need for the poison control information to be written on the tube. Baking soda is an antacid and cleanser and a pure product in a paste form. Herbal toothpastes contain healing and nutritional substances that can be absorbed into the child's body.
- Remind your child that massage of the gums is important. Do not be afraid of bleeding gums. This occurs with these conditions. If gum massage is done regularly, the tissue will heal accordingly.
- Rinse with sea salt or baking soda solution or herbal mouthwash frequently to control the bacterial level.

These illnesses can be a cause of early onset of periodontal disease, but not in the majority of cases. Children who are healthy have little tartar and strong bone development. With a healthy environment and proper oral hygiene, your child will develop into a "healthy tooth candidate" with solid bones and gum support. Children must develop good hygiene habits early on, so that these habits will already be in place for them as adults.

Helpful hint: Check your child's teeth, looking for dark spots on the teeth and/or swollen gum tissue.

The Teen Years

When your child becomes an adolescent, don't let him or her start neglecting the teeth and gums! Teenagers have poor sleep habits and diets; they often eat high amounts of sugar and usually have little time to eat a well-balanced diet. Fast-food meals are not nutritious for a young adult. Living this kind of lifestyle can lead to gingivitis, an upset in the flora of the mouth that leads to bleeding gums and loose gum tissue. If not attended to, it can cause periodontal disease.

Adolescence is a time when many children get braces. If your child is wearing braces, provide special (electric) toothbrushes for him or her to work around the brackets. An oral irrigator, which will cleanse around the gum line, can be very helpful here. Otherwise, braces can make it difficult to access the gum line area. Nourish your child's gum tissue during this time with natural herbal rinses and toothpaste. It is better if your child swallows natural toothpaste than toothpaste that is loaded down with chemicals. Bacteria love to seat themselves on top of children's braces, and the simple movement of the teeth facilitated by the braces can cause the gums to become loose and spongy. Using natural products will improve this condition and make your child feel better.

12

Now You Can Reverse Gum Disease Naturally

Summarizing the Contributors That Can Lead to Gum Disease

The key problems that can create the onset of gum disease lie strictly with each individual. Simply speaking, you must develop good oral hygiene habits at an early age. If this hasn't happened yet, then I hope my book will help motivate you to develop good oral hygiene habits. Don't wait till your mouth becomes a serious problem. Gum disease comes on quietly, but like a volcano, it can erupt quickly. Here are some of the causes of gum disease that you should try to eliminate in your life.

Fear

This can be the number one cause of gum disease. Years ago dentistry was, well, in the Dark Ages. I remember the days when I had to raise my hand to tell the dentist that the drill was hurting me. He then would stop drilling. Today there is a myriad of anesthetics such as Novocain and laughing gas (nitrous oxide). You can also learn to meditate—a process I myself use when receiving dental treatment. Learning pain management can help you to heal. Pain may be your number one fear, but pain is only there to assist you: it signals a problem in health. Pain can also stimulate the adrenal system and send the blood cells to the area for you to heal. It is the shocking pain or unannounced pain that we are truly afraid of. If you trust your dental professional and feel in control, you will never fear a slight pain sensation. Be sure to talk to your professional, and let him or her know you are fearful, as he or she will try to help.

Neglect

This takes two forms: lack of at-home care and lack of professional care. If you neglect to do proper home care (oral hygiene) through simple laziness, or have never been shown how to work properly on your mouth, then you probably have gum disease. Start reversing the process of gum disease *now*, by using the proper products with the right amount of knowledge and discipline. Second, a lack of professional care can lead to gum disease. Having your teeth cleaned only every three years is not enough! A good, thorough cleaning should be done two or three times a year, and may be needed more frequently. Don't be lazy about it. Make cleaning your mouth a priority, and schedule an appointment today!

Denial of Problems

If we deny the problems and symptoms of gum disease they will not get better, but worse. Follow the steps in the previous chapters to find a quality professional, and remember: home care in dental hygiene is 90 percent of the cure! So start the process and work on your mouth. Besides, worry, which is tied to stress, only exacerbates the poor condition of the mouth. And don't forget, denial of problems only postpones the inevitable, and conditions will persist and get worse if not attended to.

Poor Selection of Dental Professionals

If you are not comfortable with your dental professionals, then change your dentist or hygienist. Do not stay with a professional with whom you are not comfortable. Proper selection is important in establishing your desire to continue with their services. If you are comfortable with your dental professional, then you will return frequently as needed. Frequent check-ups and ongoing maintenance as provided through your professionals are very important.

Improper Home Care Regimen

Dental products are not magic in and of themselves. You must work with the healing nature of your mouth, and some products are better than others. Natural products will nurture the gum tissue and help you keep the gum tissue tight and healthy. You want the gum tissue to lie flat against the tooth to eliminate pockets that can develop, because pockets are holding areas for food and bacteria. Bacteria sitting under the gum next to the tooth can create bone loss and loose tissue.

Do more than remove plaque from your teeth—also nurture the tissue. The pockets of the gums must be cleansed and at the same time the gum tissue should be nurtured with natural products so that the tissue lies flat against the tooth structure. A healthy tooth has a proper bone support with healthy gum tissue.

Lack of Finances

If it is a lack of money that is troubling you and keeping you from confronting your gum disease, then think of a way to fund the removal of the problem, even if it means going on a payment plan. Speak with your professional to work out a payment plan. The result is a natural reversal of gum disease without worry.

Diet

If your diet is high in sugar, then you are encouraging bacteria to thrive. As a reminder, sugar turns to acids in your mouth. If you have acidic saliva, then you are more apt to have free excess calcium in the mouth. If free acid arises in the mouth, you will then develop chronic gum inflammation, which will lead you to gum disease. To reverse this pattern, try to reduce your sugar intake. I have noticed that people who drink large amounts of coffee have a larger tartar buildup in their mouth. These people especially build up tartar in the glandular area on the lower anterior teeth. If I look into a patient's mouth and notice a lot of plaque or calculus, loose teeth, or receding gums, I realize that the pH of the mouth is not balanced. Neutralizing the pH can be done with sea salt rinses. You can also use baking soda as a buffer to balance the pH of your mouth. (Litmus paper can be used to test the acidity of your saliva.)

Starchy foods tend to stick on teeth and leave a film. If you do not remove the film, then plaque and tartar will develop. Brushing with massage and a cleansing toothpaste will help eliminate this problem. Following the cleansing routine, you must nurture the gum tissue and feed the new cells that are brought to the surface with gum massage.

Menopause Problems

Many women in menopause realize that something is happening to their smile line. What is the smile line? The gum line or outline of your teeth. If you notice that you are now getting a "long-in-the-tooth" appearance, it may be due to menopause. If your gums are loose and spongy, then this might be due to a hormonal problem. Your gums may bleed more readily and your tissue will start to recede. The most important thing is to moderate your diet. As the aging process starts and the hormones change, we must work with a healthier diet.

Cut out any or all refined sugar in your diet. Turn to the natural sugars that you find in fruit. Most important, eliminate caffeine and alcohol. Do not eat cultured dairy products, because they can create a habitation for bacteria in the mouth. Drink plenty of water, as it will help you to balance the pH of your saliva and flush the acids out of your system. Use supplements such as vitamins and minerals, and use natural products. Herbs with natural vitamins and minerals are great in juices for a quick jump start in the morning. You can take a multiple vitamin, but remember that eating a balanced diet has priority over supplementation. You are what you eat! Try not to eat too many spices, because they can cause the gums to get irritated. If you like spices, neutralize the heat in your mouth by cooling it down with alkaline foods.

Diseases

Certain diseases can contribute to gum disease. (See chapters 2 and 11 for more information.)

Anemia

Anemia is a condition that reduces red blood cells and can cause the onset of gum disease.

Herpes Simplex

Herpes simplex is a virus that affects the tissues of the mouth. This condition may be chronic and stay latent in the mouth and may appear later on in life.

Lichen Planus

This is a chronic condition related to the immune system. It can affect people later on in age.

Pemphigus

This condition of the skin and mucous membranes affects elderly people, and women more frequently than men.

Alcoholism and Tobacco Addiction

Oral effects shown in alcoholics and smokers are reflected as gum disease.

Cancer of the Head and Neck

Cancer of the head and neck can cause gum disease.

HIV (AIDS)

People with HIV have oral manifestations that appear as inflamed gum tissue. They may also suffer from an unpleasant mouth odor.

Leukemia

Gum disease is a problem here because of the immunosuppression of the disease.

Medications

The most common culprits are:

- Antiseizure medications for epilepsy—Dilantin
- Drugs for multiple sclerosis—cyclosporine
- Prolonged antibiotic therapy
- Antihistamines
- Anticholinergics—atropine, scopolamine, propantheline
- Antihypertensives—guanethidine (Ismelin) and clonidine (Catapres)

Children and Gum Disease

If your children are poorly motivated and do not want to take care of their teeth, this can lead to future gum disease. Prevention is the best method of reversing gum disease. Thus a fun and playful hygiene home care station is a necessity in your bathroom. If your child has his or her own bathroom this can be easy to implement. If you have to share the bathroom, then create separate hygiene stations. Allow each child to have an area that is his or her own. Lighting is very important, and if you can find a good magnifying mirror, this might help your child see the back of his or her teeth. Have music available so that you and your family can brush and massage your gums with rhythm.

Motivating Your Child

Poorly motivated children are candidates for gum disease. You are their guardian to help them prevent the onset of the disease. Highly motivated children have highly motivated parents; those who continue to work with their own hygiene problems help to motivate their children. Make sure to compliment or reward your child for good oral hygiene, and compliment your child's smile. As just discussed, set up a fun and playful work station: help your children love their teeth by using fun products such as:

- the new innovative electric children's brushes in fun shapes and colors
- a water pick
- good-tasting natural toothpaste
- music to make your children happy and help them increase dexterity and rhythm

Also, keep these considerations in mind when selecting a dentist/hygienist for your child:

- Select a good pedodontist and/or a general dentist who likes to work on children.
- Look for a clean, cheerful office where the professional emphasizes the *prevention* of tooth decay and gum disease.
- Choose a quality dentist and hygienist who are proficient in teaching good oral hygiene.

The cleaning of a child's teeth and gums can be looked on as a way to further his or her total body health. Motivate your children early on in their development.

Now that you've read the book, remember these important tips:

- *Diet:* Examine your diet. If you are not eating correctly, then try a high-protein diet, eating more vegetables and more protein-rich foods. Stop consuming lots of sugar in your diet. Eating a high-sugar diet will cause the plaque to build up with bacteria. Make sure to eat three balanced meals a day, drink plenty of water, and stay away from breads and processed foods. This will help you to elevate your immune system while you're in the process of reversing gum disease.
- *Vitamin supplements:* Take a multivitamin supplement every day. Try taking Cal Max (which is liquid calcium and magnesium) or calcium that you can metabolize well. Take a vitamin C pill (in addition to your multivitamin). Vitamin C is needed for collagen buildup of the gum tissue. (However, as ascorbic acid

can burn the tissue, it may be better to take vitamin C in pill form.) Take a magnesium supplement. It is an important catalyst because it assists in calcium assimilation. Think about taking phosphorus, which makes up one-third of the bones and teeth. Note: If you are taking antacids, you may be deficient in phosphorus. Check with your medical doctor to see if you are iron deficient. If so, take iron supplements.

As you move forward to eliminate gum disease from your life, remember to:

- Set up a room with accessible dental products.
- Have a strong daily routine that becomes second nature.
- Use scented products that taste and smell great, such as mint-flavored baking soda toothpaste and echinacea toothpaste.
- Floss first, then brush massage the teeth and gums to loosen particles from the teeth and gums.
- Use an oral irrigation system with herbs or peroxide under the tissue.
- Brush and tone with a soft toothbrush and with a gentle massage action.
- Last, check your smile in a mirror. You should look and feel great!

Appendix

Resources for Natural Products

The following is a list of Web sites and chain stores through which you can obtain some of the products mentioned in this book. Feel free to e-mail me at toothfairyshow.com for questions pertaining to any of the products and store locations.

Baking Soda Toothpaste (Arm & Hammer)

Web sites

www.ChurchDwight.com

www.drugstore.com

www.eckerd.com

Chain stores (among others)

Kmart

Walgreens

Bioforce Echinacea Toothpaste, Oral Rinse, and Spray

Web site

www.BioforceUSA.com

Chain stores (among others)
> Fresh Fields
> Whole Foods
> Wild Oats

Herbal Tinctures

Web sites
> www.wilner.com
> www.quantumherbalproducts.com
> www.northamericanherbs.com

Oral Irrigators

Web sites
> www.waterpik.com
> www.drugstore.com
> www.eckerd.com

Chain stores (among others)
> Brandsmart
> Cheaper by the Dozen
> Kmart
> Longs Drug
> Target
> Walgreens

Peelu Toothpaste

Web sites

www.bnnatural.com

www.nhe.net

www.magicgarden.com

Weleda Toothpaste (Calendula, Plant Gel, Myrrh, Salt Toothpaste)

Web site

www.Weleda.com

Chain stores (among others)

Fresh Fields

Whole Foods

Wild Oats

Bibliography

Alternative Medicine. Fife, Wash.: Future Medicine Publishing Group, Inc., The Burton Goldberg Group, 1993.

Jensen, Bernard. *Foods That Heal: A Guide to Understanding and Using the Healing Powers of Natural Foods.* Garden City, N.Y.: Avery Penguin Putnam, 1988.

Perry, Dorothy A., R.D.H., Ph.D., Phyllis L. Beemsterboer, R.D.H., Ed.D., and Edward J. Taggart, D.D.S., M.S. *Periodontology for the Dental Hygienists.* Philadelphia: W. B. Saunders Company, 1996.

Rateitschak, K. H., E. M. Rateitschak, H. Wolf, and T. M. Hassell. *Dental Medicine,* 2nd ed. New York: Thieme Medical Publishers, Inc., 1989.

Senzon, Sandra, R.D.H. *The Hygiene Professional: A Partner in Dentistry.* Tulsa, Okla.: Penwell Publishing Company, 1999.

Stay, Flora Parsa, D.D.S. *The Complete Book of Dental Remedies.* Garden City, N.Y.: Avery Publishing, 1995.

Index

Index

Index

Index

Index

Index

Index

sea salt rinses, 21, 23, 61
seaweed, 31
sedum, 134
seeds, *see specific types of seeds*
selenium, 131
serotonin, 74
sesame seeds, 31, 90
Shiatsu massage, 77
shoulder stand (yoga posture), 71
signs of gum disease, 9–13
　bleeding gums, 11–12
　gum abscesses, 12–13
　halitosis, or bad breath, 10
　malpositioned teeth, 10
　receding gums, 11
silicon, 131
sleep, 23
Smith, Dr. David, 14–15
SmokeEnders, 55
smoking, 39, 55–56, 124, 188
sodium lauryl sulfate (SLS), 82
somatic pain disorder, 60–61
sonic scaler, 18
Sparine (promazine), 38
spicy foods, 22
staphylococcus, 94
steroids, 33
stevia, 137
strawberries, 91
streptococcus, 94
stress, 41–56, 97, 120
　alcohol and, 54–55
　bruxism and, 45–47
　cheek biting and, 48
　chronic, and gum disease, 42–44
　essential oils for, 98
　gum chewing and, 49
　ice chewing and, 48–49
　lemon sucking and, 52–53
　methods for reducing, 69–79
　mind-body-spirit connection, 44–45
　nail biting and, 51–52
　positive, 43
　thumb sucking and, 51–52
　tobacco smoking and, 55–56

　toothbrush abrasion and, 53–54
　vitamin deficiencies and, 51
sugar, 42, 74, 82, 120, 172, 186, 187, 191
sulfa drugs, 127
sulfur, 131–32
sunflower seeds, 90
surgical removal of gum tissue, 16–17
Swedish massage, 76–77
sweets, 22
　stress and eating, 50–51
synovial fluid, 64

Tai Chi Ch'uan, 78
tartar, *see* calculus ("tartar")
tea bags, soothing pain with, 61, 62, 65
teas, herbal, 135, 136
tea tree oil, 75, 137
　toothpaste, 88
teen years, 183
teeth:
　energy relations of, with organs of the body, 102–107
　grinding and clenching of, 43, 45–47
　malpositioned, 10
　minerals affecting, 128, 130
　tooth wrap, 155–56
teething, 66–67
teething rings, 67
Tegretol (carbamazepine), 38
television referrals to dental professionals, 166
tennis, 72
therapeutic healing, 101–19
　defined, 101
　electric toothbrushes, 116–18
　energy relations of teeth with organs of the body, 102–107
　flossing, 114
　from hygienist, 107–108
　mouthwash, 115
　oral irrigator, 111–13
　personal oral hygiene and, 108–109

Index

About the Author

Sandra Senzon, R.D.H., an entrepreneur and author, has worked in the world of dental hygiene for twenty-six years. In 1989, as an educational tool for new patients, she created the Tooth Spa, which offers a softer approach to dental hygiene. She writes, hosts, and produces a weekly cable television show for children called *The Tooth Fairy Show*, which advances dental hygiene and oral care. She is also the author of five children's books that motivate children to care for their teeth. She has lectured before state and local hygiene associations, and is the author of *The Hygiene Professional: A Partner in Dentistry*. She also has been published in *The Farran Report* and *Dental Economics*. She has traveled as far away as Japan as a guest of a toothbrush company to select products for that company. Sandra Senzon's dental practice is located at 200 Madison Avenue, Suite 2201, New York, NY 10016. She can be reached at 212-684-1844 or e-mail at SSenzon961@aol.com. She can also be reached via her Web site, toothfairyshow.com.